KABALISTIC HEALING

Kabalistic Healing

SHIRLEY CHAMBERS

KEATS PUBLISHING

LOS ANGELES

NTC/Contemporary Publishing Group

Library of Congress Cataloging-in-Publication Data

Chambers, Shirley (Shirley A.)
    Kabalistic healing / Shirley Chambers.
        p.   cm. – (Healing wisdom)
    Includes bibliographical references.
    ISBN 0-658-00644-4 (pbk.)
        1. Cabala—Health aspects.   2. Health—Religious aspects—Judaism.
    3. Mysticism—Health aspects.   4. Spiritual healing and spiritualism.
    I. Title.   II. Series.

    RZ999 .C43 2000
    615.8'52—dc21   00-043571

Published by Keats Publishing
A division of NTC/Contemporary Publishing Group, Inc.
4255 West Touhy Avenue, Lincolnwood, Illinois 60712 U.S.A.

Managing Director and Publisher: Jack Artenstein
Executive Editor: Peter Hoffman
Director of Publishing Services: Rena Copperman
Managing Editor: Jama Carter
Project Editor: Claudia L. McCowan

Text design: Laurie Young

Printed and bound in the United States of America

International Standard Book Number: 0-658-00644-4
00 01 02 03 04 VP 18 17 16 15 14 13 12 11 10 9 8 7 6 5 4 3 2 1

To Babaji . . . the beginning

CONTENTS

CONTENTS

viii

Contents

FOREWORD

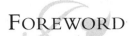

Whe I was asked to write the foreword for Shirley Chambers's book on healing and the Kabalah, I immediately jumped at the chance. I knew this was an opportunity for me to organize my thoughts about the mind/body problem that has fascinated me for years. A book such as this on spiritual healing and its implication of healing at a distance must ultimately face the same problem.

As a scientist, it is extremely important to have a model and mechanism that explains the phenomenon that we observe. This holds true for spiritual healing as well as more traditional healing involving allopathic medicine. It is precisely this rational and mechanistic approach that has allowed modern medicine to make such great advances. What I find most intriguing about this book is the model of the Tree of Life. The Kabalistic Tree of Life is an ingenious glyph that provides a model for a spiritual explanation of the mind as well as consciousness, and just as the periodic table in chemistry explains chemical reactions, the Tree of Life can explain the mechanism of miracles. Contained within this complex model is the structure of our physical world as well as our mental world and higher worlds. Perhaps Shirley Chambers's greatest contribution is her explanation of how these different worlds interact through overleaving of Trees representing each world.

This comes at an important time in present-day medical research. Some of the most exciting research in medicine today is in the neural sciences and cognitive psychology. Dynamic imaging with MRI (magnetic resonance imaging) and PET (positron emission tomography) has revolutionized our theories of how the brain forms images and stores memories. Recent landmark works such as *Descartes' Error*, by neurologist Antonio R. Damasio, and *Philosophy in the Flesh*, by philosophers and linguists George Lakoff and Mark Johnson, give neurological mechanisms that can explain emotions and feelings in terms of "body states" and concepts being shaped as metaphors of bodily projections.

Traditional medicine at this time supports the theory that the mind is not separate from the body. It has good evidence that the mind is, indeed, embodied. This seems to preclude the idea of a collective mind or a higher self, and presupposes it is actually neural processes that we experience as the mind. It is the orthodox view that having a mind means that the organism forms neural representations, which can become images and are manipulated in a process called thought. If we were to continue in this trend, medicine would be inextricably grounded in materialism with no room for spirit, a higher self, or a soul.

If we agree not to disagree violently, the mind/body problem could be elegantly resolved with new understanding made possible through this book. The Kabalah and the Tree of Life support and incorporate the orthodox view of neuronal complexes, body states, embodied metaphors as concepts and thoughts, and the sum total of visceral actions as feelings. These are all represented on the Tree of Life in the Worlds of Assiah and Yetzirah. In these Worlds are contained the physical body, including the brain and all its reflexes. This is the level in which the behaviorists and now the cognitive psychologists are working. Their methods and results have irrefutably proven themselves over time. Basically, this has given us the conscious mind and the unconscious mind. There is no place for the superconscious mind in this conception. Yet what is lacking in this point of view and in orthodox research is the definition of the "listener." This listener cannot be self-created and included in a loop of feedback brain centers or body centers. Damasio inadvertently traps himself in many pages of his book by referring to this aspect of mind without defining it. In so doing, the need for a higher mind becomes evident. This need is fulfilled in the Kabalah by the superconscious mind.

Ultimately, everything is energy contained in form of some sort. When we speak of mind being disembodied, we do not mean mind without form. We simply mean that the information of the mind is contained in another state of energy as signals are contained in radio waves or other frequencies in the electromagnetic spectrum. The Kabalah teaches that this state of pure energy contains information, which we can call mind on some level. Out of this is the physical universe created. Recent research in particle physics confirms the possibility of this proposition. New experiments at CERN, the European laboratory for particle physics near Geneva, demonstrate that there is a state of pure energy called "quark–gluon plasma." This was the state of the universe immediately following the Big Bang from which all matter came. The most fundamental building blocks are quarks held together by gluons derived from this plasma.

Healing of any kind is ultimately dependent upon the body healing itself. Whether a medication is given, or surgery is used to remove tissue or bring tissue together, the final step in the healing process is inherent in the body's own immune and inflammatory response. All methods of healing are simply triggers to bring this natural response about. The placebo response is just as legitimate as radiation therapy or chemotherapy in the treatment of cancer if it causes the tumor to regress. What makes a good doctor or healer is his skill and knowledge of the healing mechanism. The more precise the treatment the better is the result.

I have personally witnessed physical cures that cannot be explained by known medical mechanisms. I have seen breast tumors disappear in front of my eyes. I have seen a diseased heart instantly restored to normal in its rate and rhythm through a healer's hands. These miracles are no longer miracles if understood within the context of Kabalistic healing and the Tree of Life.

Descartes's famous statement, "Cogito, ergo sum," "I think, therefore I am," has led us down the reductionist path of a deterministic universe created by a detached God who set the machine in motion, and which has been diametrically interpreted by different philosophers and researchers of consciousness and the mind/brain problem. The question of the mind is whether it is extrinsic or intrinsic. Undoubtedly, the correct answer is that it is both, just as the question of whether God is immanent or transcendent is also in the answer that He is both.

With this understanding in mind, Kabalistic healing can be understood and appreciated for its tremendous organizational contribution in many fields. It allows us to understand our physical bodies, our psychology, and our interconnection with each other through our collective superconsciousness in a rational and scientific manner.

As a medical student at the University of Michigan in 1969, one of the favorite phrases that was used throughout my early training was that medicine is an art, not a science. We knew that a good physician was more than a mechanic. What we termed art was really spirit. This phrase will always be true, but with the information in this book, we can convert this art to a science, and make room for more art.

—WILLIAM BAUER, M.D., M.S.

extrinsic or intrinsic. Undoubtedly, the correct answer is that it is both, just as the question of whether God is immanent or transcendent is also in the answer that He is both.

With this understanding in mind, Kabalistic healing can be understood and appreciated for its tremendous organizational contribution in many fields. It allows us to understand our physical bodies, our psychology, and our interconnection with each other through our collective superconsciousness in a rational and scientific manner.

As a medical student at the University of Michigan in 1969, one of the favorite phrases that was used throughout my early training was that medicine is an art, not a science. We knew that a good physician was more than a mechanic. What we termed art was really spirit. This phrase will always be true, but with the information in this book, we can convert this art to a science, and make room for more art.

—WILLIAM BAUER, M.D., M.S.

ACKNOWLEDGMENTS

I acknowledge with gratitude . . .

Eric Sprung, who formulated the diagrams, input the text, and edited the prepublication manuscript.

Vicki McDermott, Arlene McClure, and Brent Schwarz, teachers and friends who are the core around which the Karin Kabalah Center continues to expand.

Ruth Wall and Bill Lane, who have always been there for guidance and a helping hand.

All former and present students at the Karin Kabalah Center, who provide the structure for the continued evolution of the mystical tradition of the Kabalah.

INTRODUCTION

Kabalistic healing is complex, for it comprises two distinct subjects, Kabalah and healing, that combine to produce a very potent synthesis. The applications and techniques of Kabalistic healing are as varied as the spellings of the word *Kabalah*. Although the applications may vary, however, the principles involved are essentially the same. To know and integrate these principles, and to learn to use them effectively, is the responsibility of those utilizing Kabalistic healing. Just as there are over-the-counter medications as well as those that are available only with a prescription from a medical professional, there are both personally and professionally directed uses of the principles (medications) of Kabalistic healing.

To understand Kabalistic healing, we must understand the meaning of the word *mysticism*. The intangible flow of will/intent contained in the words of Kabalistic teachings enables one to become the reality of his existence. The American Heritage Dictionary defines mysticism as "immediate consciousness of the transcendent or ultimate reality of God." We have all read about the mystics of the past, those individuals who seemed to have a close contact with some higher power, most often defined as God, and whose lives were dedicated to that power, often at great personal cost. Kabalah reveals a living God, a power of life that expresses into the physical world and its experiences for the purpose of its own empowerment. This power has been described since the beginning of time, and has been worshiped and often feared in many different time frames, cultures, and states of consciousness. Mankind's relationship to this power has not been to its reality, but rather to the various forms in which it has been contained and expressed.

The expression of this power is through principles, which are brought into the physical world through mankind's activities and experiences. This power itself is balanced, harmonious, and whole, only seemingly becoming imbalanced and distorted when expressed through activities inappropriate to the beauty of its expression. The most common name for this power is "God." God, then, can be said to be the life-will, the intent for existence, expressing itself through multidimensions and multiforms. Nothing can exist without this mandate of life-will; therefore, there is nothing that can be said not to be God. And yet, as we see imbalance and distortion, both physical and emotional, existing in our world, it becomes difficult to believe that everything truly is God.

One often sees many different spellings of the word *Kabalah*. The beginning letter of the word seems to have evolved from "c" to "q" to "k," the most common today. It was once thought that "c" related to the traditional form of Kabalah, "q" to the hermetical or ritualistic form, and "k" to the mystical. The spelling of the terms applicable to the study also vary. Being universal in nature, each class or group of individuals studying Kabalah adapts it to their culture, language, and level of awareness. Perhaps the variety of spellings might also indicate that the essence of Kabalah and its teachings is of at least equal if not greater importance to the form it establishes. Although the form is important in that it contains the essential concepts, it is the essence contained within that form that impacts the inner nature of mankind. If one is dying of thirst, he does not refuse to drink water because he does not like the design or color of the cup!

We can perhaps better understand this incongruity by comparing this great life-will power to a principle of force within our physical world: electricity. Although electricity is a powerful force that can be used to either cure or kill, it is neither good nor bad. The results of its use or expression, however, can be defined as either.

Perhaps the best way to define mysticism as it relates to Kabalistic healing is as the level of awareness needed in order to apply and prescribe certain principles (medications) necessary to achieve balance or attain wholeness within the life experience. It is similar in principle to the level of awareness attained by a physician that empowers him to treat patients and prescribe healing remedies. This awareness comes with the achievement of spiritual adulthood, whereby one realizes the Divine flow within. It is this realization that enables one to practice Kabalistic healing with utmost proficiency.

Another way to understand mysticism is through a mundane example such as the taste of an orange. Everyone knows what an orange tastes like, yet who can explain it in words? Still, the realization of the taste of oranges is what makes us want to keep eating them. What the mystic tastes, in effect, is the Divine flow of life-will; his realization of that taste allows him to apply that flow to himself and others in order to aid in the creation of proper and balanced "life recipes." Just as an improper ingredient in a recipe results in a dish that does not taste good, improper ingredients in our lives result in disharmony and disease.

In this book you will find the words *consciousness* and *awareness* used frequently; at times, they will appear to be interchangeable. Consciousness is what results from growth, and all growth is educational. Upon completing the fourth grade, a child has the consciousness earned from that year as well as from his entire life experience up to that point. Experiences may fade from memory, but the results of their integration enable the child to effectively live "in the here and now." Not all children who complete fourth grade, even those with similar life experiences, have the same consciousness. Some may seem smarter than others or more able to apply what they have gained from both education and experience. This difference can be said to relate to awareness, or the vibratory frequency of consciousness. This vibratory frequency is relative to evolutionary age. Just as there are members of various ages within a family, there are various ages within the family of mankind. Therefore, even though the educational experience is common to many people, those completing it are of different evolutionary or spiritual ages. Awareness gives the power of comprehension; hence those with a higher awareness or vibratory frequency will be more empowered in their comprehension and expression.

No matter the level used, Kabalistic healing techniques are quite simple. They range in complexity from "over-the-counter" prescriptions that nearly everyone can use, to techniques that require the ability of visualization and a knowledge of the Tree of Life and that enable one to direct his consciousness beyond the level of visualization to soul consciousness. Each higher level requires more effort in order to achieve a state in which the techniques relative to that level become viable. All require some knowledge of the Tree of Life; however, the highest level requires a transformative process in which the words of Kabalistic understanding containing the transcendental impetus lead to the attainment of soul, or superconscious, awareness. One becomes first a Kabalist, then a Kabalist who practices Kabalistic healing.

1

The Kabalah

Many believe that "the Kabalah" is a text or book of information, but this is hardly the case. However, it is, in a sense, a "text" of knowledge that has changed form and translation many times, adapting itself to different cultures and eras and reaching those who were capable of going beyond its form to the realization contained within it. When we reach far back to the two oldest religions in the world, Hinduism and Zoroastrianism, we find a common denominator—an essence of thought—that obviously was derived from a singular source. There is much conjecture about that source, yet does it really matter what it was? What is important is the common thread that has run through past religions and into religion as we know it today. The world has always had its sages and wise ones, who taught the younger generations through stories, allegories, and myths. Man's identity, destiny, and relationship to the world around him were couched in terms that the general populace could understand and relate to.

The old saying that there is nothing new under the sun is probably quite true, as is the statement that history repeats itself. The family units of mankind operate in cyclic spirals. Each unit builds upon and repeats the experiences of the former unit on a higher level. For example, each succeeding generation in the family of mankind has had to learn the calculation of numbers in some manner—from the abacus of ancient China to the sophisticated calculators of our time. At one time, simple arithmetic was considered the highest achievement in the calculation of numbers; now we reach to calculus and beyond. Yet, while the evolution and refinement of mathematics continues, its essence remains the same.

People have always related to a source of power higher than themselves, a source that cannot be seen but whose existence is thought to be proven by earthly phenomena, such as rain, lightning, and wind. At first, people related to this power only through the intermediary of the king, priest, or—in some cases—the king-priest. There could be no personal relationship with the higher power. As human consciousness continued to evolve, however, people began to establish their own individualism; as a result, they needed to experience a relationship with that which was formerly limited to the kings and/or priests.

Around 1900 B.C., an individual emerged who served as a source for the new cycle of spirituality, and that individual is named Abraham in the Old Testament's Book of Genesis. Some people who had reached a higher level of awareness were drawn to the new concepts of man's identity, destiny, and relationship with the world and with God. Collectively, they established a new structure in which that understanding was contained. That structure, or religion, is known as Judaism. Whether we consider Abraham to be an individual or a symbol representing a collective group consciousness, we see that a new wave of understanding had begun.

The travels of Abraham and his followers are related in Genesis. Their extensive travels—from Ur in the mountains of Chaldea, through Persia to Egypt, and then to Canaan—suggest that the concepts of this new understanding may have been synthesized from several sources, including the famed Chaldean Book of Numbers; the Zoroastrian scriptures, or Gathas; and even the Egyptian sacred volumes of the Thoth-Hermes. Even Abraham's former name, Abram, may have been derived from the same word as *Brahmin,* which in Sanskrit means "expansion." It was the Brahmins of high priestly origin who brought the origins of Hinduism into India.

By following the succession of names in biblical history, we arrive at the important personage of Moses, whose story symbolically represents the breaking of mankind's identity with its physical/sensate existence. Thus we arrive at a time when people could apply to their lives the new understanding that began with Abraham. At about the same time that Moses is said to have been leading his people into a new land, the Indo-Europeans were invading India, bringing new ideas and doctrines to that area. Then followed a very important time for mankind, during which many noted philosophers and teachers were born. From about 600–400 B.C., we find Buddha, Confucius, Lao Tse, Pythagoras, Socrates, Plato, and Aristotle, to name a few. And, in that same

3

era, we find the emergence of Merkabah Mysticism, which existed from about 538 B.C. to A.D. 70. This could be considered the source of the first written tracts in the system later to be termed Kabalah. These were known as the Heikhaloth Books, based on the first chapter of Ezekiel; some believe they were based on the first chapter of Genesis, as well. It has been suggested that the Wheel of Pythagoras and the Wheels of Ezekiel derived from a similar, if not the same, philosophy.

As mankind's history continued, he began to individualize the concepts and forms of his belief systems, otherwise known as religions. Religion has a very important purpose, for it has served as the containment for the expression of Divinity and Divine principles as they reflect to mankind the reality of his existence. Many of the philosophers and teachers who endeavored to bring mankind to a new level of understanding were rejected and, indeed, often persecuted. In his refusal to continue his growth process and take ever-greater responsibility for his life and actions, mankind began to identify even more with his external world. As new levels of consciousness were unfulfilled, distortions in the life of mankind became evident and the vices of the old level became intensified.

The next impact upon the flow of religion that would later flow into the Western world was made by the man known as Jesus—a world teacher, or avatar—who was born into a Jewish family. Members of his family were said to have been Essenes, a mystical sect within Judaism, and it is believed that during his life, there was a communicative exchange between Jesus and the Essenes. The Dead Sea Scrolls are essentially the teachings of the Essenes and contain much the same understanding we find in the mystical teachings of the Kabalah. Jesus himself stated that he did not come to abolish the law, but rather to give it a new meaning. As clearly indicated in the New Testament, Jesus often spoke quite differently to his disciples than he did to the masses—again, another indication that there are varied levels of understanding available to those who have the ability to comprehend them. This does not make one level greater or lesser than another. A second grader might be much smarter for his age than an eighth grader is for his. Within the family of mankind, it is spiritual age that makes the difference, and spiritual age is determined by evolutionary growth.

The essence contained within the mysticism known as Kabalah surfaced much earlier than the word itself, which did not appear until the twelfth century A.D. *Kabalah,* which means "to receive," connoted a mouth-to-ear transference of the higher teachings from teacher to student. The passing of time and the advent of written works, however, has enabled a greater number of people to "hear through the eyes" in receiving this understanding. The word *Kabalah* might now more properly mean "to receive the realization" of one's true identity or reality.

We must once again turn to Judaism to trace the history of what was to become Kabalah, for it finds its growth within the higher understanding of Judaism's religious texts. The Torah is the foundation of Judaism. Also known as the Pentateuch, it consists of the first five books of the Old Testament, said to have been set down by Moses. Basically, the Torah consists of rules and regulations by which Jewish life is governed; but even more important for mystics, it contains a higher understanding of mankind and his evolutionary process.

The next important text in Judaism is the Talmud, which is composed of two works, the Mishna and the Gemara; it contains the history of the Jews within a time frame of about one thousand years. The Talmud was created to enhance and expand upon the teachings of the Torah. Other important texts are the Midrash, an extension of the oral law; the Halakah, which deals with religious, ethical, civil, and criminal law; and the Aggadah, which contains theological speculation, moral and ethical teachings, prayers, philosophical discussions about man's relation to the universe, and other, more mystical, discourses. It is said that the Kabalah emerged from this tradition.

The Talmudic period lasted from about 135 B.C. to A.D. 1040, and produced two Talmuds: the "Babylonian," completed around A.D. 200–300, and the "Palestinian," completed around A.D. 300–400. The Babylonian is the larger of the two and has been studied more, perhaps because Babylon became a center of the speculative branch of Kabalism.

Kabalah itself divided into two branches. Practical Kabalism, which concerned itself with rituals designed to control energies, influenced the magic of western Europe. Speculative Kabalism concerned itself with the understanding of the higher levels of mankind and the universe, as well as the interaction between the two. The source of speculative Kabalism may be traced to the Masseh Bereshith, or "History of Creation," which later evolved into the Sefer Yetzirah, or "Book of Creation."

The Sefer Yetzirah is considered the foundation stone of the Kabalah. Although its authorship is attributed to Abraham, it is purported to have been set down by Rabbi Akiba around A.D. 100–200. However, it contains all the information set down in the Chaldean Book of Numbers, which would most likely have been previously studied by Abraham.

It has been said that the practical and speculative branches of Kabalism were united in the work known as the Zohar, or "Book of Splendor," which is said to have been written by Moses de Leon of Guadalajara, Spain, around A.D. 1280. It is a canonical text and is the only Kabalistic text to be ranked in importance with the Talmud and the Torah by the rabbinical community. It is quite lengthy, containing some nineteen parts with commentaries and discourses on many topics.

Along with the Torah, the Sepher Yetzirah, and the Aohar, the fourth major work underlying the origins of Kabalah is the Bahir, or "Book of Brilliance," which was compiled from earlier writings in Provence, France, around the last half of the twelfth century. It contains, among other topics, the theory of reincarnation, and is a connecting link between the early Gnostics and the medieval Kabalists. It is a small text, containing some thirty to forty pages, that came to light during the thirteenth century, though it is said to have been written in the first century.

By the eighteenth century, interest in Kabalism had dimmed in western Europe. Its doctrines, however, were kept alive by the Christian mystics who had become engrossed in its teachings as early as the thirteenth century. Kabalistic writers of the nineteenth and twentieth centuries made important contributions to Kabalism, with the greatest impact being made by those who continued to move forward with new understanding.

Now, rather than an informative text of understanding, Kabalah becomes a process that man can use to further the growth of his own spirituality. Just as medicine and science have

7

evolved through the centuries, the same growth impetus has impacted spirituality. This growth has imparted to mankind the ability to bring either greater balance or greater imbalance into his life. Mankind is now within reach of his potential for spiritual adulthood as well as the strength of its expression, yet in many cases, he has not developed the inner education to handle that strength. Distortion on the inner levels results in disease and distortion in the manifested world.

This brief history of the mysticism known as Kabalah illustrates that there has been and will continue to be a flow of understanding contained in many structures throughout its evolutionary life. This essence of understanding is much more potent today than it was in times past, for just as with mankind, its growth has empowered it. History shows us individuals who paid a high price when they used the archetypal principles or energies of the Kabalah for personal aggrandizement. With a great force of will, they invoked specific energies of the Tree of Life, creating a tremendous imbalance. This would be similar to opening the floodgates of a dam without having constructed proper channels for the water. Energy, like water, takes the path of least resistance, and in man, these paths would be his own weaknesses.

The study of Kabalah can be likened to the study of medicine. Although a medical student studies informative texts, that alone does not qualify him to become a physician. The texts are only part of a process of integration and application, which the medical student completes and the results of which are then demonstrated in his ability and skill in the practice of his vocation. The Kabalistic process, however, relates not to outer development, but inner. Through inner development the Kabalist is able to effect harmony into his life and, like a physician, help others. Just as there are physicians who facilitate the body's healing process, and psychologists, psychiatrists, and therapists who facilitate emotional healing, there are now those who facilitate healing from the soul level. These individuals are known as Kabalistic healers. They do not detract from the other levels of healing; rather, they enhance them as they work with the spiritual aspects of the body, mind, and spirit totality of mankind.

2

The Tree of Life

"And God said, Let us make man in our image, after our likeness" (Genesis 1:26). And then man returned the favor by creating God in mankind's image, giving God a human form and human emotions. This anthropomorphization of God was an important step in man's establishment of a personal relationship with God. But just as man comes to realize that he is more than his physical body and senses, we must now come to understand that God is also more. If, as stated previously, God is the life-will within all existence, and this life-will expresses itself through multiforms, then to arrive at a better comprehension of God we must look at the expressions of that life-will. To do this, we use the archetypal glyph or diagram called the Tree of Life.

What is an archetype? As defined by Webster's, an archetype is the "original pattern or model of which all things of the same type are representations or copies." According to Carl Jung, an archetype is an inherited idea or mode of thought that is derived from the experience of the race and is present in the unconscious of the individual. Both of these definitions apply to the Tree of Life.

The Tree of Life has been spoken of or depicted in one form or another by nearly all ancient cultures. The Tree of Life and the Tree of Knowledge of Good and Evil are mentioned in Genesis, and nearly all Eastern religious scriptures speak of a tree, sometimes depicting it as a glyph and sometimes as an actual tree. The glyph of the Tree depicts in a "blueprint" form those principles that constitute the totality of expression of God's life-will. If, as stated in Genesis, man was created in the image and likeness of God, then man was also given God's principles. Although the principles are the same, we must understand that man's expression of them—unlike God's—is limited by his mortal existence. A child has within him the same types of expression as his parents; however, they are expressed differently into his life than his parents' are into theirs.

As an archetype, the Tree of Life symbolically portrays that which manifests through all form, from an atom to the universe. Because it has been carried forward through the evolutionary life of mankind, it fulfills Jung's definition, and the glyph itself speaks quite loudly in the language of the unconscious, a language of symbolism. Because the Tree of Life is collective—that is, present in the collective unconscious of mankind—its impact is far greater than that which is personal or limited to one individual. As the collective unconscious continues to grow in strength, archetypes themselves become more powerful as well.

Figure 2.1 depicts the Tree of Life as it has evolved into present-day use. When looking at it one sees circles and lines, and spaces enclosed by the circles and lines. There are ten solid-line circles and one dotted-line circle. The highest circle, Kether, has dual aspects because the entire Tree emanates from it and returns to it. Therefore, we have ten actual (solid line) circles or spheres, yet there are twelve aspects or types of expression. As stated, due to the fact that the Tree of Life emanates from and returns to Kether, Kether has two different types of expression. The dotted-line circle, Daath, is yet to be developed within this evolutionary lifespan, yet is applicable to the lesser cycles within that span. The reason for this will be explained as we further investigate the Tree, but for now, let us identify the spheres as they are traditionally named and as they are shown on the diagram.

13

The circles or spheres of the Tree are called *Sephiroth;* the singular is *Sephirah.* They represent stages in the emanation of God or Spirit from pure existence to the physical world, each stage being one of the principles that compose the totality of the expression of life-will. The Sephiroth are numbered in the sequence of their emanations, a sequence often described as the "Lightning Flash" of creation. We might say that this Lightning Flash represents the big bang; the creation of potential, or the fertilization of the egg that, over eons, developed into our world. As this expressive emanation descended from the highest Sephirah, each subsequent Sephirah modified it in accordance with its own pattern. And, although expressing a particular principle, each Sephirah actually contains all of the principles. This would be similar to putting different colors or dyes into separated drops of

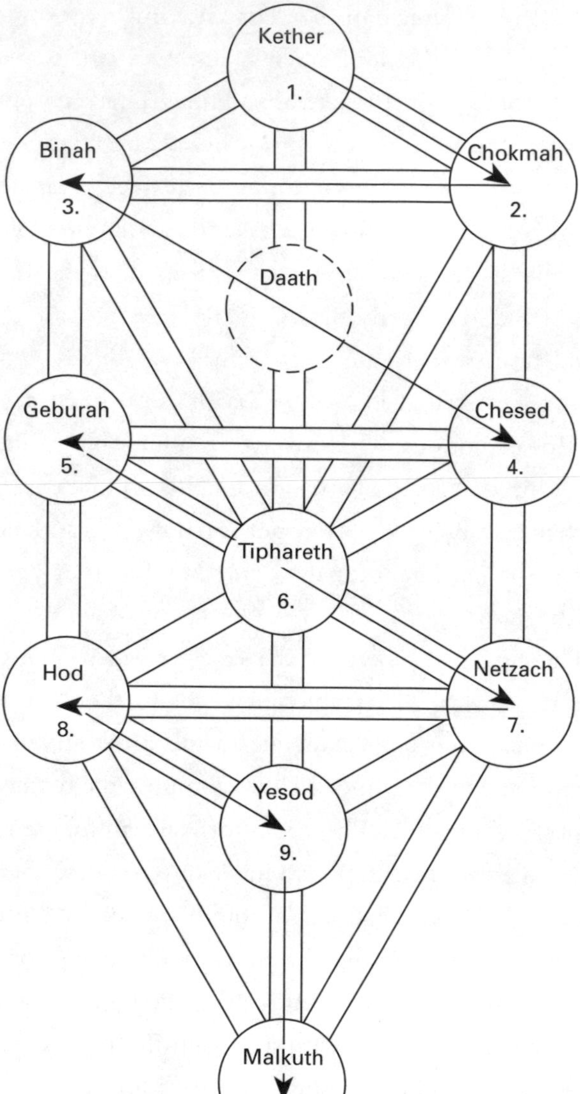

14

FIGURE 2.1. SEPHIROTH AND LIGHTNING FLASH

water. Each drop would appear different in its expression, but would still be essentially water.

The names of the Sephiroth of the Tree of Life, and their titles, are as follows:

1. Kether—The Crown
2. Chokmah—Wisdom
3. Binah—Understanding
4. Chesed—Mercy
5. Geburah—Judgment, Severity
6. Tiphareth—Beauty, Harmony
7. Netzach—Victory, Eternity
8. Hod—Splendor, Reverberation
9. Yesod—Foundation
10. Malkuth—Kingdom

The Sephirah enclosed by a dotted line is termed Daath; its title is Realization. The twelfth aspect referred to previously relates to Kether, which by virtue of its inherent dual polarity receives back that which it emanated after the emanation has completed its journey through experience.

The lines between the Sephiroth are called paths, and they indicate the use of the principles of the Sephiroth. For an analogy, we could say that one of the Sephiroth represents the principle or force of electricity; the path would represent the appliance powered by the electricity; and the spaces enclosed by the Sephiroth and paths, termed triads, would represent the result. Remember, however, that this is a very mundane analogy relating to tangible aspects, while those represented by the Tree are intangible, becoming tangible only as they are evidenced in physical existence.

Figure 2.2 depicts the Tree divided into three columns, or pillars. The right and left pillars each contain three Sephiroth in a vertical alignment; the middle pillar contains four—five, if you include Daath. Each of the three pillars represents the descent of a similar type of energy as it expresses on different levels.

The right pillar is known as the Pillar of Mercy, the Pillar of Force. The Sephiroth on this pillar all relate to levels of force. In descending order we can term these God's or Spirit's force (universal), the soul's or superconscious force (collective), and unconscious/conscious force (personal).

The left pillar is known as the Pillar of Severity, the Pillar of Form. The Sephiroth on this pillar all relate to levels of form. Again, in descending order, these are God's or Spirit's form (universal), the soul's or superconscious form (collective), and unconscious/conscious form (personal). The lowest level with which we can equate these opposites is that of desire (force) and intellect (form); however, these are actually sensate determinates of personal force and form, also known as creative power and creative ideation.

When force and form interact, they produce movement or momentum. When gasoline burns (force) in an automobile engine (form), propulsion is the result. You might say that the propulsion is the will of the automobile for its movement. The middle pillar of the Tree is the Pillar of Will, which formulates a consciousness to contain will. Another word for consciousness could be *mind*. The will of the middle pillar was previously introduced as life-will, which is the mandate for something to exist, as opposed to life-force, which enlivens existence. In descending order, there is the Will of God, or Spirit; realized mind/will (Daath), a level of growth mankind will not achieve in this current cycle, but which

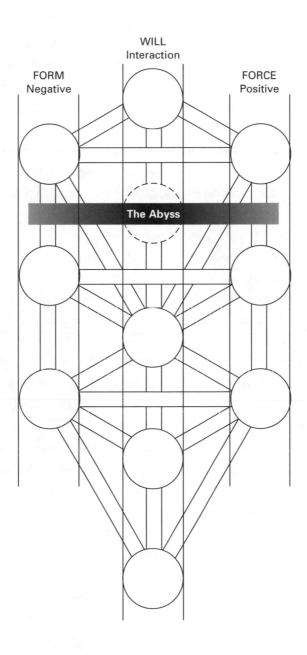

FIGURE 2.2. PILLARS AND THE ABYSS

does apply to the lesser cycles; soul or superconscious mind/will, transforming universal to collective; unconscious mind/will, transforming collective to personal; and conscious mind/will, transforming personal into manifestation or activity.

Each Sephirah on the middle pillar of the Tree has a duality of force and form with which it interacts and through the interaction of which interaction its principle of mind/will is empowered, or, in other words, grows. This is much like the force and form of experience, through which the child is enabled to grow into adulthood. Through continuous education and experience the child develops the strength and responsibility to effectively express his adult life.

The source of all existence is the life-will of God or Divinity. In order to express itself and be empowered by that expression, life-will, by virtue of its movement into existence, created its own opposite polarities. As these polarities descend in vibratory frequency, they become the dualities of existence. The Tree of Life, mentioned in Genesis and other mystical texts, is pure empowerment, pure will—the middle pillar of the Tree. The Tree of Knowledge of Good and Evil is represented by the side pillars, the duality brought into existence for the purpose of experience. Good relates to force and is free moving and expansive, but useless unless contained. Evil relates to form, which restricts and holds force and is thus considered severe. It is the darkness or solidity of form that, when impacted by light or force, reveals the splendor of Divine will as it propels mankind on his journey to spiritual adulthood or enlightenment.

In figure 2.2, you will note what is termed the "abyss." Its functions are many, but in simple terms, it represents the separation between the Creator and the created, a separation that is gradually spanned by man's own realization as he attains his status as a cocreator with Divinity. We can see a similar "gap" in the life of a human: a baby is born and there is a tremendous gap in comprehension between that baby and his parents. However, as the child grows into adulthood, that gap is narrowed, continuing to shrink until one day, even though his parents are older and have experienced a great deal more of life, the former infant relates to them as peers. The child's realization of his own growth upon each step of his life's journey helped bridge the separation between his consciousness and that of his parents.

The shaded areas in figure 2.3 are what are known as the triads of the Tree of Life. In this chapter we will refer to the traditional titles and meanings of these triads. Later we shall define them as they represent the natures of man's psyche. Each triad is composed of three Sephiroth and three paths. It is the expression of the Sephirothic principles through the paths relative to the level or world in which they exist that creates the triads.

Triad One, at the top of the Tree, is composed of the Sephiroth Kether, Chokmah, and Binah. It is known as the Supernal Triad, also called the "Supreme Mysteries." This triad points upward, indicating the singular source from which the world was emanated. Kether is the totality of the Supernal Triad, containing polarity within itself. However, in order to multiply a singular unit, it must first be divided; one times one is one. Kether divided itself into the polarity of its masculine and feminine father-mother aspects—Chokmah and Binah, respectively—which, by virtue of Kether's division, exist upon a lower level of vibratory frequency.

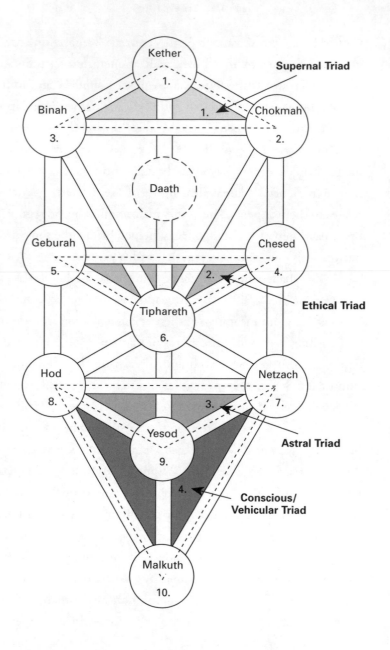

20
𝓛❧

FIGURE 2.3. TRIADS

The purpose of God's emanation of will into existence is for its own empowerment, generated through experience. Will can do nothing of itself. You may express the will to go home, but if you don't know where home is (form) and you don't have the motivation (force) to make the journey, that expression of will would be useless. In your expression of will is already contained the destination and motivation, but that doesn't get you home. You have to transform the polarity within the will into the duality of activity. Otherwise you would not get home.

Within God's will of emanation was contained the polarity of force and form, but they had to be transformed into the duality of force and form so that activity could take place. Thus one divided into two, yet still retained its own principle of will. The two therefore were active, more tangible, one might say, than the idea for them contained within the one. In order to augment itself, the one had to transform and divide so that interaction could occur.

21

Although we have divided Kether into its lateral divisions of father and mother, we refer to Kether as Father in its vertical relationship to the energies below it on the middle pillar. If this naming convention is understood to refer to polarity, not gender, one should have no qualms about using the term *Father* in speaking of Divinity. Mankind is the feminine aspect of that vertical polarity, and is growing in awareness toward his own motherhood, his own creatorship.

Triad Two is known as the Ethical or Moral Triad. Tiphareth is its focal Sephirah, and its duality is comprised of Chesed and Geburah. This triad, as well as the next two triads, point downward, directing their influence into manifestation through mankind. Each Sephirah on the middle pillar becomes feminine under the projection of will from the Sephirah above it, and projects masculine will upon the Sephirah below. The exception is Malkuth, which is form (feminine) to Kether's force (masculine).

Triad Three is known as the Astral Triad; it consists of Yesod as its focal Sephirah and Netzach and Hod as its dualities. You will note that Triad Four, the Conscious/Vehicular Triad, shares Yesod's dualities of Netzach and Hod. Triad Four represents Triad Three's projection into each life experience, and although Triad Three can be said to exist in an intangible level or frequency, it is still part of experiential existence. This will be more fully explained in the discussion of man's psyche.

In summary, force and form—and the interaction between them—result in growth momentum and the development of consciousness. Relative to the life experience, they are all that matters. Their interactions occur within four basic levels, or worlds, or four different types of expression. There are ten principles, reflecting the totality of Divine life-will, which can be expressed within the four levels or worlds. When those principles are held in balance and are developed in conjunction with each other, harmony, balance, and peace ensue; but when they are not, distortion and disease appear. It is the work of the Kabalistic healer, through spiritual counseling and the application of those principles, to help those in need begin the healing process in accordance with each individual's pattern.

3

Planes and Worlds

The previous chapter mentioned planes and worlds, and although these terms might seem similar, there is a difference between them. For example, we exist upon the physical plane of the earth, yet we see, have access to, and are impacted by the immediate universe in which our earth exists. Together, our universe and our earth are considered our world. A plane or level defines an area of activity, while a world includes that activity as well as everything that affects it, even that which is intangible.

The Tree of Life is considered a World that can be divided into four planes, each of which is contained in a lesser world upon that Tree. There are four Trees of Life comprising our Universe, each containing four lesser worlds or subworlds, which relate to the planes. The planes within each Tree, from the highest level to the lowest, are termed spiritual, creative, emotional/

intellectual, and physical. The subworlds in which these planes exist are termed atziluth, briah, yetzirah, and assiah, also in that same order. The initial letter of the titles of these subworlds is not capitalized, since the four Worlds comprising the Universe are also entitled Atziluth, Briah, Yetzirah, and Assiah, each of these containing four subworlds entitled atziluth, briah, yetzirah, and assiah.

Figure 3.1 depicts the Tree of Life with its plane and subworld divisions, the planes divided by solid lines and the subworlds shown as circles. Nothing in the universe is separate; on the contrary, everything is interconnected. What happens in our lives and in our world impacts all existence like a ripple effect. In figure 3.1, you can see that the physical plane is influenced by a subworld that encompasses the lower half of the Tree, including three Sephiroth of life-will. We could also call this life-will "intent." The next two higher planes, the emotional/intellectual and creative, are also influenced by three Sephiroth, or principles of life-will/intent. You will see, however, that the highest plane, the spiritual, is encompassed within a half-circle that contains only two Sephiroth upon the middle pillar. This is because there are four Trees of Life that make up our universe, and since nothing is distinct and separate from that in which it exists, these Trees and what they symbolize are interrelated and interactive. Due to the overlaying of the four World Trees, the third or highest Sephirah of the highest subworld is found in the next higher World, thus forming the link between the highest subworld in a lower World to the lowest subworld in the next higher World.

The four Trees that comprise the Universal Planes of existence and were emanated by the Divine are entitled the World of Emanation (Atziluth), the World of Creation (Briah), the World of Formation (Yetzirah), and the World of Manifestation

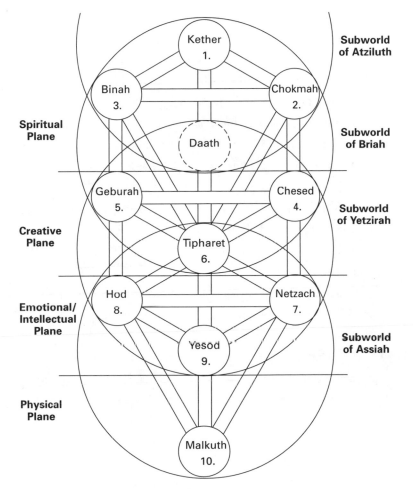

Spiritual
Plane

Creative
Plane

Emotional/
Intellectual
Plane

Physical
Plane

Kether
1.

Binah
3.

Chokmah
2.

Daath

Geburah
5.

Chesed
4.

Tipharet
6.

Hod
8.

Netzach
7.

Yesod
9.

Malkuth
10.

Subworld
of Atziluth

Subworld
of Briah

Subworld
of Yetzirah

Subworld
of Assiah

25

FIGURE 3.1. PLANES AND SUBWORLDS

or Activation (Assiah). These are the emanation of the life-will, or intent, of God establishing its dual polarities and extending outward into increasingly dense levels until reaching the limits of its expression in what we see as physical existence, depicted in figure 3.2. We could place a World Tree in each of these four Universal Planes. The highest of the four Worlds, Atziluth, is the Spiritual World, also called the Archetypal World and the World of Emanation, wherein God divided the principles of the Universe. It is the World wherein God said, "Let us make man in our image, after our likeness . . . ." (Genesis 1:26).

Who is the "us" that God is speaking to? They are the Elohim, those Divine principles of pure force, yet a patterned force that is projected into the next lower World forming the pattern itself. The principles of the Sephiroth in Atziluth are assigned "God names."

The next World is Briah, the World of Creation. Here the force of Atziluth is contained into the pattern for the Universe, as formulated by the patterned force of Atziluth. Held in this World is what we could call the "perfect plan," the ideal reality that both the universe and mankind are striving to attain. This is the creation spoken of in Genesis 1:27: "So God created man in his own image . . . ." The principles of this World are personified as archangels.

Yetzirah is the World of Formation, also known as the World of the Psyche and the World of the Minds. In this World the force of Atziluth and the patterns of Briah produce their off-spring, man and his world. In Yetzirah, thought forms are a reality and ideas are clothed in electric and magnetic matter. "And God said" expresses the thought within the mind of God that

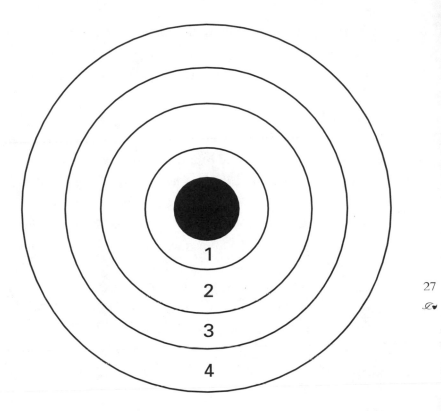

1. Spiritual World—Emanation

2. Creative World—Creation

3. Emotional/Intellectual World—Formation

4. Physical World—Activation

FIGURE 3.2. CREATION OF THE PLANES

resulted in the creation of the universe. Since man was created in the image and likeness of God, it follows that as man matures, he also creates with his thoughts. Genesis 2:7 states, ". . . and the Lord God formed man." The principles in the World of Yetzirah are personified as angels.

The final World in the emanation of the Universe is the World of Assiah, or the World of Manifestation, Demonstration, and Action. It is what we call our physical world, comprised of both seen and unseen elements—physical matter, subatomic particles, atoms, molecules, particles, and waves. This World contains solids, liquids, gases, and the four ethers: chemical, life, light, and reflecting. It is the World of the physical vehicle we call mankind, as well as the senses that enable that vehicle to function. The principles in this World are described as the energies of the planets of our solar system. Thus we have a way of defining those principles as they are to be expressed into our world. Just as the infant matures into adulthood, mankind—through his educational life experiences—matures into a level of godhood. Genesis 1:14 states, "And God said, Let there be lights in the firmament of the heaven to divide the day from the night; and let them be for signs, and for seasons and for days, and years."

The Divine forces in Atziluth form spiritual principles and creative patterns in Briah, which are then instilled in their potentiality within man in Yetzirah to be manifested into experience upon each level of growth through mankind in Assiah. In order for one World to flow into the next, there must be interaction, and that interaction occurs as the lower half of a higher World is placed over the upper half of the next lower World, ensuring a continued flow to and from the Godhead—not only within each

World but in the Universe itself. This interaction or overleaving is depicted in figure 3.3 in which the four World Trees are shown placed upon the Universal Tree. You will note that the upper half of the highest World Tree extends above the Universal Tree, this upper half consisting of three principles of life-will. In Kabalah these principles relate to "the veils." In Kabalistic terminology these veils are called Ain, Ain Soph, and Ain Soph Aur; they relate to what we might call the Cosmic Trinity: the Cosmic Father, the Cosmic Mother, and their offspring, the Cosmic Son, who in turn became the Father of our Universe. Again we see the one becoming two and the interaction of the two producing an off-spring. There is much more to this understanding, but for now let it indicate the fact that even what we consider our Universe is a part of something greater, something that cannot even be defined within the limits of the human brain. For the purpose of Kabalistic healing it is necessary only to understand the con-tinuous flow of Divine life-will that extends through all Worlds and planes.

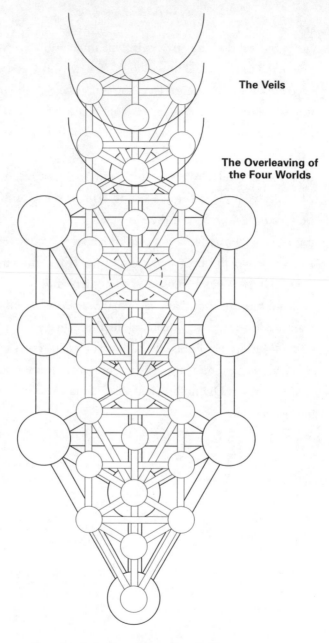

The Veils

The Overleaving of
the Four Worlds

FIGURE 3.3. THE UNIVERSAL TREE

4

God the Father, God the Mother, Man, and Mankind

Just who, or what, is man? The word *man* is derived from the Sanskrit root word *manas,* meaning mind. Since man is created in the image and likeness of God, then much as an infant is similar to his parents, man has within him God's life-will, or mandate to exist. Being pure force, this life-will coalesces into a living form through which it can express and experience. Thus man is a mind being, an aspect of life-will existing within a vehicle termed the mind. The totality of existence we call consciousness or mind exists within an intangible world and needs a vehicle through which it can experience the tangible world. Man therefore creates a vehicle in his image and likeness, and we call that vehicle mankind. Thus mankind is manlike, created in the image and likeness of the consciousness that contains and transmits its force of intent and pattern to its vehicle.

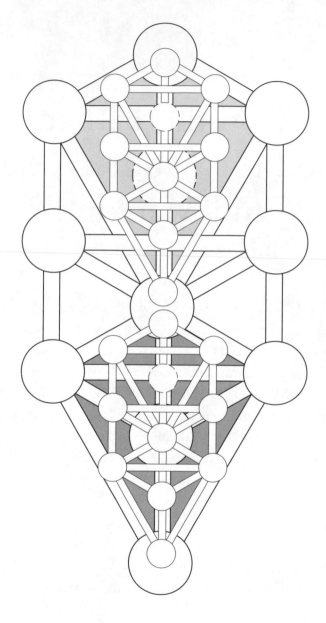

FIGURE 4.1. THE TREE WITHIN THE UPPER AND
LOWER HALVES OF EACH TREE OF LIFE

We know that God's principles of force exist in the World of Atziluth, the World of their emanation. These God principles are created into patterns of form in the World of Briah. Therefore, we see God's consciousness in Atziluth and God's "body," or vehicle—comprised of the patterns for the principles of God's expression—in the World of Briah. These two Worlds can be said to be the Worlds of the Creator, the Father, who through a vertical expression of Himself creates his own masculinity (Atziluth) and femininity (Briah). The offspring of that union, seen in the World of Yetzirah, is man, the mind-being of consciousness who is born an infant and by virtue of his evolutionary growth toward maturity is destined to achieve a godlike state where he can express Divine principles appropriately upon the level of his own awareness. Mankind, the vehicle through which man expresses those Divine principles inherent in his own being, is created from and experiences within the World of Assiah.

We have only four Trees, two of which we regard as God's Worlds and two as man's Worlds, yet both God and man express the principles of the Tree through four Worlds. In each of the four Worlds we can place an entire Tree of Life within both its upper and lower halves. This gives us four lesser worlds within God's Worlds of Atziluth and Briah, and four lesser worlds within man's Worlds of Yetzirah and Assiah. This placement of a Tree of Life within each half of the Tree is depicted in figure 4.1. Within each World Tree the upper half is considered force, while the lower half is form for that force; thus we could say that each World contains an intangible and a tangible half. Remember too that the halves are not separate, but exist one within the other. We are depicting in two dimensions something that is multidimensional, much

33

like a blueprint. When working with the Tree, however, we use it without the placement of Trees within each half, but with the understanding that each half of the Trees of God's or man's Worlds represents one of the four Worlds.

Figure 4.2 depicts the Worlds of God and man, the shaded areas indicating the lesser worlds contained within the four Worlds. Those areas not shaded are areas of transformation between those worlds, or the force and form halves, of each Tree. Interaction occurs within each World, as well as with the Worlds above and below each World; this interaction is depicted in figure 3.3. You will note from figure 3.3 that the lower half of each World Tree overlays the upper half of the next lower Tree. God's active world in the World of Briah therefore overlays and interacts with man's spiritual world in the World of Yetzirah. As they relate to the four greater Worlds, God's Worlds are Spiritual and Creative (Atziluth and Briah), while man's are Formative and Active (Yetzirah and Assiah). God expresses His creation, and man formulates and activates it. Man, the mind-being in Yetzirah, who is created in the image of God in Atziluth, should formulate into Assiah—the world of mankind—the likeness of the body of God's principles in the World of Briah. When these principles are not expressed in accordance with God's pattern, as that pattern is relative to each stage of man's growth, then disharmony and disease occur, reflecting imbalance and distortion in man's creation. A teacher presents the principle of the calculation of numbers to the student, but if the student errs in the application of the principles, the fault lies with the student, not the teacher or the principle. The resultant incorrect answer indicates that something has gone awry. When one understands the beauty of

34

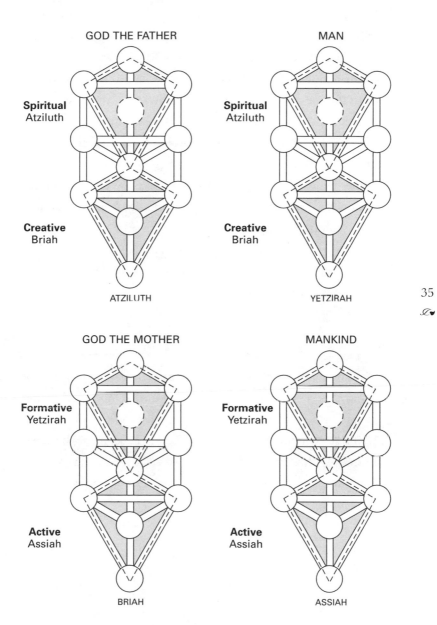

GOD THE FATHER

Spiritual
Atziluth

Creative
Briah

ATZILUTH

MAN

Spiritual
Atziluth

Creative
Briah

YETZIRAH

GOD THE MOTHER

Formative
Yetzirah

Active
Assiah

BRIAH

MANKIND

Formative
Yetzirah

Active
Assiah

ASSIAH

FIGURE 4.2. GOD'S WORLDS AND MAN/MANKIND'S WORLDS

Divine flow and the potential of its appropriate expression, one can see that distortion occurs when the flow has become disrupted or distorted within man's worlds. The flow is constant, cycling to man and back to its source; however, the flow has its channels in the belief systems of man. Quite often it is diverted into inappropriate channels and wasted; sometimes the flow is dammed up, in which case it ultimately bursts forth with extreme pressure, creating havoc and disasters. To understand this flow and the principles of its expression is to begin to understand Kabalistic healing.

The next step is to understand the makeup of man, the mind-being of consciousness, whose continued growth develops and empowers those Divine principles with which he has been endowed. Man is a creative and spiritual being whose reality is depicted by the World of Yetzirah. The World of Mankind, Assiah, represents not only the vehicle through which man experiences, but also the physical and formative, or sensate, world of his existence. The vehicle we call mankind is composed of the elements of the earth upon which he exists. When the vehicle dies, those elements return to the earth, while man, the consciousness within that body, projects himself into a new vehicle to continue the evolutionary growth process in the seemingly never-ending cycles of time.

5

The Functions
of Man

The Sephiroth, or Centers, of the Tree of Life represent not only the principles of Divinity as they relate to each World, but also the functioning aspect through which each particular principle is normally expressed. In Kabalistic healing, it is important to understand these functions as they relate to both man—the mind-being—and mankind, the vehicle through which man experiences the physical world.

Figure 5.1 is the blueprint for man, that being of consciousness that is comprised of force (expressive) and form (creative) aspects, with the expressive contained within and activating the creative.

Although man's functions are assigned to the Sephiroth, the paths connecting them determine their use. Man's functions develop what are termed "natures," depicted by the triads outlined

38

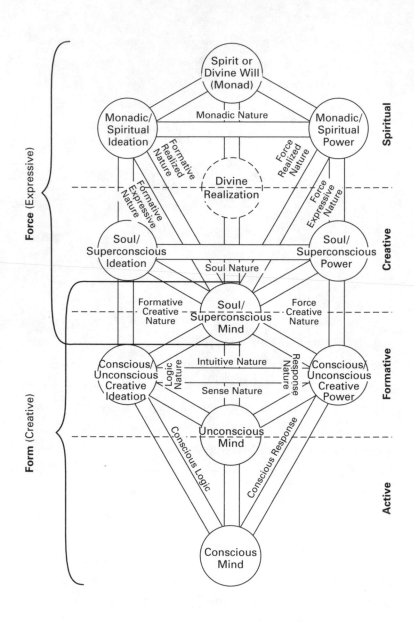

FIGURE 5.1. THE WORLD OF MAN (YETZIRAH)

by the Sephiroth and paths. The nature of someone or something is its inherent character or basic constitution. A nature qualifies existence: the nature of a rose is to bloom; the nature of a dog is to bark; the nature of an artist is to paint. Just as with the Worlds, which contain subworlds, there are greater natures in which many lesser natures are contained. A dog expresses an animal nature, but within that greater animal nature lies his nature to bark.

Because God created the Universe, it is obvious that God's nature is to create. Made in the image and likeness of God, man's innate nature is also to create, and create man does, on every level of his existence. For creativity to occur, there must be expression that contains the idea, thought, or intent for that which results. God first had an idea for His expression before it became contained within His creation, just as artists have a pattern for their expression before they create it on canvas. Man, therefore, has these same expressive and creative abilities, portrayed in figure 5.1 by the upper and lower halves of the Tree of Yetzirah. These abilities, as they relate to levels of activity, are designated by the triads within those halves. The use of any ability or nature strengthens and perfects it; thus, the use of man's expressive and creative abilities strengthens and perfects man— in other words, enables him to evolve or grow. Throughout growth, man creates his image and likeness into mankind, the vehicle for man's experience.

Just as in school, growth in life should be a balanced continuum. History, English, mathematics, geography, and so on should be learned at a common pace, appropriate to the student's grade. If one of these subjects is not integrated, the student is kept from moving into the next grade. The failure to integrate

39

all the subjects creates a distortion in the balanced continuing education of the student. When distortion or disease becomes evident within the body of mankind, it indicates that something is amiss in the evolutionary educational growth of the consciousness of man. What is usually amiss is the integration of man's educational subjects—those subjects relating to the principles of the Tree as they apply to man's growth, or evolutionary educational process.

For any expressive or creative activity, the three aspects that make up the Tree of Life are necessary: force, form, and interaction, or will. In order to create a painting, an artist must have the motivation, the idea, and, most of all, the intent or will to express his idea. As he applies his nature, or ability to paint, the artist strengthens that ability. As his ability is strengthened, the artist's work reflects this, since it too improves.

Man's "canvas" is mankind and its world. Man's artistry improves as he becomes more godlike in the expression of his inherent potential, a potential that contains the principles of Divine intent and the capability of expressing them into the beauty and harmony of his world. Perfection is relative to each stage of growth. A fifth grader achieves perfection when his studies reach the highest level attainable at that level. This entitles him to enter sixth grade, then seventh, and so on, until the student completes all the education necessary in order for him to express his chosen vocation. Man's vocation is that of a creator, but in order to achieve that status, there needs to be the educational process, which we call "life." When that educational process is completed, man will not leave life, but will live it to its utmost in beauty and harmony. Kabalah teaches a living God, one that man expresses through his being into the beauty of life experience. God did not create the life experience for man to escape from, but rather for him to live in. What man needs to learn from life experience relative to his spiritual age, or what is distorted or incorrect in what he has learned, reflects itself into mankind. This reflection is called "disease," or "dis-ease," a lack of ease or harmony.

When you examine figure 5.1, remember that the upper half of the Yetziratic World of man is force, or expression, and the lower half is form, or creation. Since each World contains four subworlds, then the spiritual and creative subworlds that occupy the upper half of the Tree constitute the spiritual world within the totality of man/mankind, as represented by the Worlds of Yetzirah and Assiah. The formative and physical subworlds, or levels, on the lower half of this Tree make up the creative world within that totality. These subworlds, or planes, are designated in figure 5.1 by dotted lines. You will note that these lines extend through the centers of the middle pillar Sephiroth, which become transformers between the levels directly above and below them.

In Genesis, the Spirit of God moving upon the face of the waters represents God's intent which subsequently brought the Universe into existence, as well as its dualities of force and form. The movement of the principle of intent, or will, draws back to that which expressed the intent, the results of the experience that was established by that intent. The intent of a child is to learn. To learn, the child must apply the dualities of intellect (form) and motivation (force). Through the application of intellect and motivation, the child acquires knowledge. This knowledge relative

41

to a certain type of expression can be demonstrated in the child's life. For instance, if that knowledge applies to science, it would then develop or enhance the scientific nature of the child. Man acquires knowledge as a result of his participation within his life experience, through which certain lessons are studied and the knowledge derived from them applied to the various grades of evolutionary life through which he grows from infancy to maturity.

As in life, the child of God is born as an infant, and becomes ever more aware of its Divine inheritance as it matures. The infant stage of man is symbolized by the lowest Sephirah on the Tree, Malkuth. The various stages of growth to be achieved are depicted in the area of the Tree between Malkuth and Kether, the highest Sephirah on the Tree. Each of the Sephiroth on higher levels of the Tree represents a higher stage of man's will and his acquisition of knowledge within levels of his educational growth. These major stages, indicated by the middle pillar Sephiroth of Yetzirah in ascending order, represent the aspects of man's mind, the awareness of which increases as man evolves. Mankind is born into and experiences within the tangible world in a physical body. Without it he could not function in the world. Yet the consciousness which directs mankind's activity in the physical world is that of man, who, although intangible to the physical senses, also has a physical level of expression, the conscious mind. It is through the activity of the conscious mind that man "grows," or evolves. Mankind's physical body is made of flesh and blood, while man's physical body can be said to be a body of creative consciousness. How these respond to and interact with each other will be explained later. For now, we are studying the makeup of man.

It is easier to understand the evolutionary life of man when we compare it to a physical lifetime and its growth cycles, which is why we use the physical lifetime as an analogy.

To summarize what we have covered to this point, man is a spark of Divine life-will containing in potential the principles of his source. Man's life-will, like God's, by virtue of its movement (growth), develops its dual aspects of force and form as they relate to each level of growth. Man's growth also develops the knowledge of the use of those principles, first to continue his educational development and then to express his vocation as a creator. Man's growth is ordained by Universal nature, just as the physical body's growth is ensured by the nature of the physical world. One need not direct the body to grow; it will do this automatically as long as it is provided with proper nourishment. It is through man's experiences that he obtains the nourishment needed for his growth, but it is Universal nature that indicates the pattern for the stages of this growth. Just as the strength of the physical body increases with growth, the intellect and motivation that direct that body develop accordingly. A man with the strength of a thirty-year-old and the intellect and motivation of a five-year-old can cause great harm to himself and others around him. Such a person creates disease and distortion in the world of mankind. We cannot stop the growth of man's strength of will any more than we can stop the growth of mankind's body. The will of Universal nature ensures its development, whether or not we are aware of it.

The densest and lowest level of life-will upon the Yetzirah Tree of Man is the conscious mind, Malkuth. As all aspects of growth continue, this mind develops greater strength that enables it to contain and activate all the higher levels of the mind's development. Remember that there is only one mind, which at this time is divided into three aspects or levels of growth, first contained in potential, but which then blossom into existence as evolutionary education develops them. The conscious mind exists within the physical level of the creative world of man. As you will see in the overleaving of the Trees representing man and mankind, the conscious mind is the will that directs the vehicle called mankind in its activities. As illustrated in figure 5.1, the conscious mind uses logic and response paths that join it with its principles of creative power and ideation to experience the world of existence, the physical world.

44

As Einstein stated, force can be neither created nor destroyed; consequently, the life-will as expressed from God (the Creator) through man (the created) cannot be destroyed; it can only be transformed. This transformation occurs through growth within the form of activity. Thus life-will, the essence of man, continues, and therein lies the concept of reincarnation, a concept often misinterpreted. Mankind dies at the end of each allotted lifetime, the elements of the body or vehicle returning once again to the level from which they were derived to form the body. Consciousness, however, contains life-will at its core, and does not die but continues on into a new "day" or lifetime, formulating a new vehicle in which to experience. The individual we identify as ourself, the form that is our conscious existence, does not continue; however, the consciousness that took unto itself that form, and then discarded it, does coalesce another form. The conscious mind that served the former vehicle died along with the vehicle. However, what that conscious mind developed continues to exist with each subsequent expression into existence, building a new form that will develop a conscious mind for its lifetime based on what has been gained from all lifetimes in the past. That aspect of life-will which has been developed by the conscious minds' experiences through all previous lifetimes is called the unconscious mind, earlier termed by psychology as the subconscious mind.

It is important to understand the unconscious, because in it are accumulated the reactions to past experiences, reactions in a form of knowing. This reactive knowing is not intellectual or intuitional, but instinctive. The unconscious has achieved its growth as a result of all the experiences in which the conscious minds of all lifetimes have participated, experiences designed by Divine intent to enable man to grow from the infancy to the maturity of his existence. The unconscious can be likened to a computer; what you program into it is then projected by it upon certain key-ins. The language of the unconscious is one of symbols. Sometimes these symbols connect with certain experiences and produce neurotic reactions, which are reactions that are more intense than an experience or situation calls for. Something within a present situation provokes a response equal to the sum total of all past responses by consciousness to similar situations relating to the same principle, although not necessarily to the same type of activity. The unconscious is very complex, and it is not the purpose of this book to present an in-depth understanding of it; however, a basic understanding is necessary in order to comprehend Kabalistic healing. Unless the consciousness of the healer is able to rise above the level of the unconscious, all healing energies are brought forth through the will/intent of the

45

unconscious and its containment of "knowledge," which can and often does pattern healing energies.

You will note that the unconscious mind draws upon the same functional principles of creative power and ideation as the conscious mind. The conscious functions of these principles, represented by the Sephiroth, can be seen in all creative activity. A newborn baby believes himself to *be* the world into which he is born, but he gradually comes to distinguish himself from that world. As the child develops his sense of identity, he begins to express the potential of that identity into his world. His world, while at first very small, expands only as he achieves the strength and responsibility to actively participate in it. Freedom equals responsibility, and the maturation process should grant both in equal amounts.

In the infancy of man's growth, he too identified with his external world, as well as the intangible or expressive aspect of that world, the physical senses. This was the involutionary arc. It was necessary for man to identify with mankind so that through mankind's experience, man could begin to establish his own identity and his own individuality by learning what he was not, just as the infant begins to learn that he is not the world around him. Just as we say that the child develops a personality as he grows, man develops a personality as he grows, a personality that continues through all lifetimes of evolutionary growth. Man, however, has grown beyond the involutional stage—wherein he identified with the external world, expanding his consciousness within it—and is now evolving, contracting his consciousness to the core or heart of his true identity: man, the mind-being. Throughout the growth process of infancy and childhood, the unconscious has gained strength and empowerment. The unconscious principle of will is represented by Yesod—whose title, you will recall, is the Foundation—because the unconscious mind is the foundation upon which all life experiences are built. The unconscious can only empower creativity, however, based upon the concepts it has acquired throughout its growth process, concepts that were appropriate for man's infancy and childhood consciousness but which become inappropriate for an adult. Therein lies the crux. Man desires the freedom of expression of a godlike authority, but has not accepted the mature awareness and responsibility that comes with such authority; consequently, distortion, chaos, and disease are prevalent in our world. The will of the unconscious has become very powerful, its power derived from the continued growth of the universal nature that directs the growth of man, while the concepts upon which the unconscious bases its creative activity are outdated and no longer appropriate for life as man. These concepts are not intellectual but expressive. The concepts are expressed through activity, but the activity does not define the expression any more than an appliance defines electricity.

In reality the conscious mind, relative to evolutionary growth, relates to the infancy and childhood of man; the unconscious mind to adolescence and early adulthood; and the next higher aspect of the mind, superconscious, to adulthood and its expression. The evolutionary timetable for man indicates that the level of the mind to which man should now aspire is superconsciousness. What is known as the soul is the life-will within man as it draws to itself knowledge relative to its level of superconsciousness. However, man's "knowing" lags behind the empowerment of his creative strength, resulting in distorted life experiences. A child experiences life continuously integrating all that will be valuable to his experience as an adult. Certain experiences that are important for the child at certain ages are forgotten, yet the knowledge gained from them is important to his growth from stage to stage. While the unconscious mind draws to itself the results of all experiences, good and bad, the superconscious mind is nurtured only by that which is in accord with the Divine plan. This is why the Sephirah of the superconscious mind, Tipareth, is entitled Beauty or Harmony. When something is beautiful or harmonious, it is in balance and there is no distortion, chaos, or disease.

48

Jung called this principle of superconscious will the Self; it is also called the Christ Consciousness. It is the level of consciousness demonstrated by the Avatar Jesus, a level He averred that man must attain in order to find the peace that passes understanding. You will note that it is placed in the center, or heart, of the Tree of Life, for it represents the heart center within man. Just as the physical heart keeps the body functioning, Tiphareth's will/intent extends to all of the principles on the Tree, either directly or indirectly. The soul or superconscious mind develops its own duality of force and form, or power and ideation. As the heart of the Tree, this Center transforms the expressive upper half of the Tree (force) into the creative lower half (form). It translates expression into creativity.

In the overlaying of the Trees, the principles of power and ideation relating to the heart of each World remain unaffected. They stand alone, indicating their autonomy in their World. Regarding man and the world of his psyche (Yetzirah), superconscious power and ideation are reflected into and empower their perfection through the power and ideation of man's creativity, which should establish beauty and balance into the life experience. If superconscious power and ideation were developed enough to empower their reflection onto a receptive power and ideation of man's creativity, emotional and physical disease would not be as prevalent as it is today.

6

The Natures of Man

Man's creative ability—his creative structure—is made up of four natures. Jung stated that man is quaternal in nature. This reflects the four basic types of expression inherent in both the universe and man. These natures are sense, logic, response, and intuitive. The intuitive and sense natures relate directly to each other, with the intuitive nature higher on the Tree, while logic and response can relate to either or both sense and intuition. This creative structure is also composed of four principles: superconscious will, creative power, creative ideation, and unconscious will. By virtue of its placement the superconscious directs creative power and ideation, while the unconscious draws from them based upon the concepts that have been programmed into it, whether the concepts are appropriate or inappropriate to harmony in man's life. For example, a teenager often has—and should have—different priorities than an adult does; when an adult continues to act as a teen, a problem occurs.

The evolutionary experience has brought about the development of man's sense nature, which is analogous to the adolescent nature. Basically, man's logic and response are based on what his senses deem appropriate for his life. Jung stated that the development of the intuitive nature has been the goal for man. Jung's individuation of the Self can be placed upon the Tree as the journey from Malkuth, the conscious mind, to Tiphareth, the superconscious mind, or Self. The intuitive nature relates to man's adult status. Intuition is not guidance from some outside source; it is man's inner tuition, the results of his inner development acquired from the teachings of life. We could say that intuition is the inner knowing that enables one to function in the world as a spiritual adult, having all aspects of one's creative functioning in balance.

The sense nature is important for the functioning of mankind, the vehicle through which man experiences. The senses define the outer world, but they should not define or control how man reacts to what he senses. If they do, then man is subservient to the world over which he was given dominion. The process of the maturation of man is to develop the inner knowing upon which his logic and response natures are based and to gradually achieve dominion over the sense nature. When this occurs, the sense nature is empowered and in adulthood becomes free to express itself fully in the world.

In Kabalistic terms, the creative quaternity within man is called the personality. It is the personality that projects into each life a reflection of itself as an experience gatherer for that time.

Remember, however, that the four natures are not separate and distinct. Each is contained within the other, from the densest vibratory frequency to the highest. We separate them only for the purposes of identification and understanding.

The personality quaternity is developed through man's educational journey from infancy to maturity, where it then serves the adult or mature expression of man. In order to express as an adult, one must have developed the ability to do so. Before man can express his spiritual adulthood, he must develop the fourth aspect of his personality, the intuitive nature. It is through this nature that superconscious will transforms Divine patterns into man's creativity.

Although the superconscious mind joins man's creative and formative levels, its dual aspects of creative power and ideation lie within the creative level. By the will of the superconscious, or the soul, these principles transform Divine power and ideation to those same principles within the personality of man. Soul will and its force and form principles form what is called the soul nature, also known in its relationship with the personality as the individuality. At this time, the soul nature is not quaternal, but one day it will be, if man continues his evolutionary growth. This soul nature, the individual uniqueness of each Self, will direct the activities of the personality and man's creativity. The state of this condition could be considered the "promised land."

Man was not meant to live in pain and sorrow. In order to live in harmony, however, man must serve the common good. His personal world must be compatible with the collective good to which his soul has access. The collective good, in

53

turn, must be compatible with universal good. The cells that make up each organ in man's body must work together to benefit the functioning of that organ, and all of the body's organs must work together to ensure the health and welfare of the body. It often helps to think of man as a cell within the body of the Greater Being we call God. Each cell fulfills its proper pattern or function, the cells work together in the group they belong to, and the groups work together to establish bodily health and balance.

Through the realized natures of the creative and spiritual levels of man's psyche, the soul recognizes—upon each stage or cycle of growth—the goal, as well as the journey necessary to attain it. The soul will impress the pattern of that journey into man's creativity, if it is allowed to do so. However, unless man has developed those Divine principles within himself relative to each stage, and unless he has prepared himself to accept and follow a higher will than that of the unconscious, his life will not exhibit balance and harmony.

This has been a brief discussion of man's psyche and the principles and natures that it comprises. To be effective, the Kabalistic healer must thoroughly understand these aspects, and must have developed them within himself through such a transformative process as the Kabalah. Also through that process, he must have achieved the ability to raise his consciousness to the level of the soul or superconscious. This is the highest level of Kabalistic healing to which one can aspire. There are conscious and unconscious applications of Kabalistic healing, which will be discussed in this book and which can be used by those familiar with the Tree and its principles. The difference between conscious and unconscious applications is akin to that between over-the-counter medications and those prescribed by a physician. Both are effective, but just as with the physical body, professional advice should be sought when a more thorough understanding is necessary.

7

The World
of Mankind

Just as with any vehicle, the vehicle called mankind should be respected and cared for, and man, the builder and operator of that vehicle, is responsible for it. Figure 7.1 depicts the force and form aspects of mankind upon the Tree of Life in Assiah, the Manifested or Active World. This is not a lesson in anatomy, but rather an understanding of mankind and its principles and functions as they relate to the Tree. Like the body of man's psyche, the body of mankind has the same principles as man, but they are expressed relative to the world in which the physical body exists.

There is a great similarity in the World of Assiah between the body of mankind and those of the other kingdoms. The bodies all have essentially the same structures, the difference being their refinement in accordance with the consciousness that inhabits each body. Each kingdom—mineral, plant, animal, and mankind—contains the same principles developed and expressed

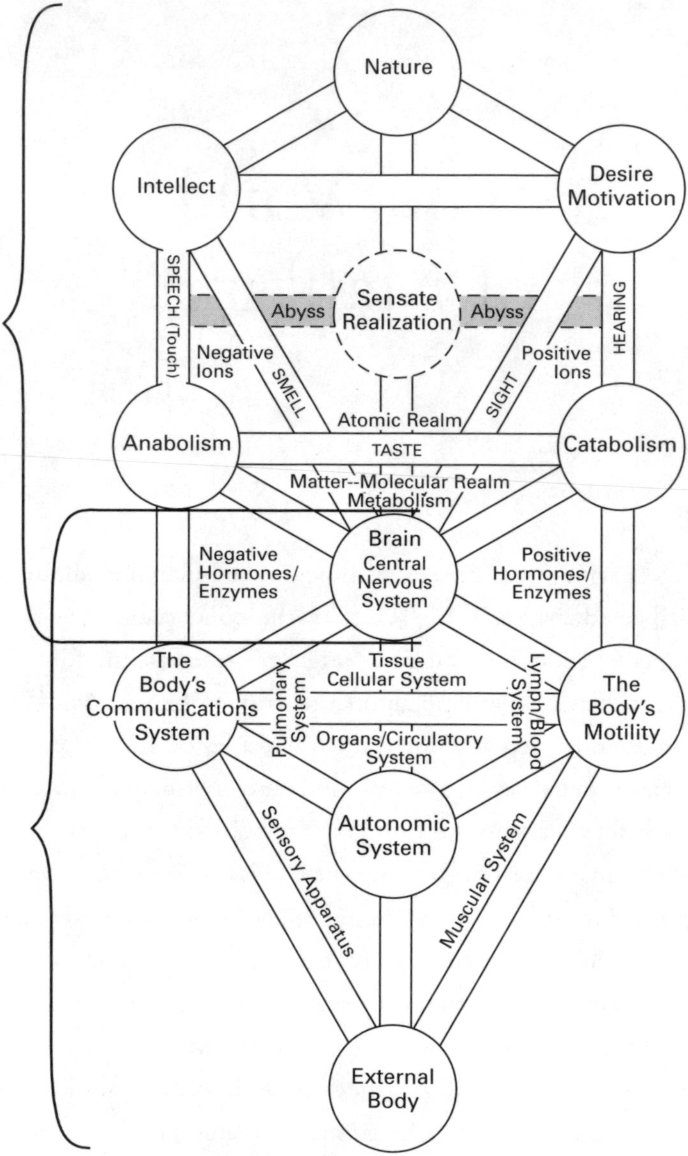

FIGURE 7.1. THE WORLD OF MANKIND (ASSIAH)

in accordance with its stage of growth. It is also important to understand that each kingdom has been built upon the experience of the kingdom below it. Thus man's experience through his vehicle of mankind was based on a consciousness developed by the animal kingdom, which gave man his "fight or flight" instinct. Man then refined that instinctual nature into his intellectual nature; he will further refine it into his intuitional nature.

The World of Mankind, Assiah, has its force and form halves. The upper half of the Tree is the intangible level, which contains the physical senses. It is also the realm of particles, waves, atoms, ions, and molecules. The highest aspect of power and ideation in this world represents the refinement of the instinctual nature into desire/motivation and intellect. It is important to remember that desire and intellect belong to the functioning of mankind—we could say that they are the operating system for the vehicle that man operates, and although they are important to that vehicle's operation, it is man's creative power and ideation that drive that vehicle.

The lower half of Assiah represents the body itself, as well as all tangible form. One can see how the three lower centers of will in this world correspond to those same aspects within the higher world of man. Malkuth, the lowest principle, which in man's world is the conscious mind, becomes in mankind's world the principle of the external body. Yesod, the next higher principle, represents the will of the autonomic system. Like the unconscious mind of man, the autonomic system reacts, but its reaction keeps the body functioning without man's continual conscious direction for its expression. We do not have to tell the heart to beat, the lungs to breathe, or the cells to function. The

59

principles of force and form relating to the physical body are its motility and its communications system, which serve both its internal and external structures.

The core of the world of mankind is the brain and central nervous system, and that principle of will in this world, as in the higher world of man, is a transformer and translator between the intangible and tangible halves. The soul triad, or individuality, of the physical world is metabolism, with its polarities of catabolism and anabolism.

Let us use an example of just how well this world operates within itself and follows directions from man's mind. (Although this example involves a sequence of events, they happen almost simultaneously.) A man's mind formulates the thought that he intends to run. This thought is directed through motivation and intellect into the brain and central nervous system, which then draw upon the aspect of catabolism to release the energy stored in cells in order to effect running. Man does not have to describe running to the body each time he wishes to run. It is already programmed into the autonomic system of the body, so when directions from the brain to the body express through the body's motility and communications system, those principles are used to enliven that pattern as well as provide just the amount of life-force needed to keep the body running until it is directed by the mind to stop.

The body must have a realization of itself in order to function properly. It must realize the unconscious mind from the higher world of man, and it must realize its own aspects of desire and intellect so they can be used by the brain. The highest aspect of the World of Assiah, like the highest aspect of every World, is the God of that World; in Assiah, we term that God "nature." It is interesting that in the World of Assiah, mankind is feminine (receptive) to the next higher World. Assiah contains the force world of Yetzirah into its form, and that totality becomes feminine to God's masculinity. As stated previously, mankind is the feminine aspect of God in manifestation. And, in referring to nature, we often use the term "Mother Nature."

The creative triads of Assiah are composed of hormones and enzymes, which are messengers directing the quaternal nature of the body's personality, comprised of the organs/circulatory system, the pulmonary system, the lymph/blood system, and the tissue cellular system. Balanced interaction must occur among these systems in order for the body to function properly.

61

The upper half of the World of Mankind, the intangible half, contains those expressions we call the senses. These must also be realized by the body in order to be used either voluntarily or involuntarily. The senses exist in man's formative world, otherwise known as the emotional/intellectual world. This world is also known as the Astral World, the world of delusion and illusion. Why is it so termed? Because the senses can deceive. What looks good and often even tastes good might be deadly to the body. This world, however, is very important, since it contains the substance from which man creates his external world. The body is part of that external world, as are the senses.

This brief description of the world of mankind is for the purpose of understanding how man, the mind-being, creates and affects that which he has created, including mankind. The next chapter will show the relationship between the worlds of man and mankind as they overlay and interrelate with each other.

8

The Principles
of Divine Expression
Reflected
Through Man

We have already discussed the functions of man/mankind as they relate to the Sephiroth, or principles, on the Tree of Life. Now we will investigate the principles that are appropriately expressed through those functions, principles that make up the body of the being called man. These principles, or essences, can only be understood upon their corresponding levels and not as they actually come into existence from their source, God. The principles inherent in man within the entire span of his evolutionary life are twelve in number; but relative to this span, they are ten, the remaining two to be developed as man continues his evolutionary growth. On the lesser cycles, however, we do consider the entire twelve. As an example, Tiphareth represents the state of spiritual adulthood to be achieved at this time; however, adulthood is not the end of one's life. In fact, adulthood is empowered by man's continued experience within it. It could be said that adulthood contains the potential for a greater realization of itself as adult growth continues. And when transition from this life occurs, what has been gained in consciousness continues into the next life experience—not in the same activity, but within an empowered awareness as a result of the former activity.

Following the aphorism "as above, so below," Divine principles are symbolized by the planetary bodies. Astrology, a science that uses the placement of these bodies to symbolize the principles of man's life, has been shown to be effective and reliable. Again, we can no more define the principles of God's expression than we can the taste of the orange, but we can define the results of their expression as qualities. Qualities then can be redefined through their appropriate (positive) or inappropriate (negative) impact. Just as electricity is a principle that can be used to kill or cure, Divine principles depend on the quality of their expression to result in either harmony or disharmony. Therefore, we can define each expression as it relates to man. But remember that the planets we see do not beam energy to Earth and man; they are symbols for the principles that come from within man as he continues developing the potential with which he was born. And, just as one relates differently throughout the ages of his life, the expression of these principles will change relative to each level of growth. The principle itself does not change, only the results of its expression. A two-year-old's perception of the world is very different from that of the twenty-year-old he becomes; even though the person's innate abilities are the same, they would be seen to evidence themselves quite differently at the two ages. The same occurs between spiritual ages. This is why it is important for astrologers to know where an individual stands in evolutionary growth before they can define the planetary influences impacting that individual's life. The stars (planets) impel; they do not compel. They can be said to be similar to a weather forecast. You cannot change the weather, but you can determine your reaction to various types of weather.

Figure 8.1 depicts the Tree of Life with its planetary representations. When the glyph of the Tree first appeared many centuries ago, Neptune, Uranus, and Pluto had not yet been discovered. When they were discovered and placed upon the Tree, their qualities fit perfectly those principles that had been assigned to the Sephiroth. Because Kether, the totality for each World, both emanates creation and receives the results of experience within it, it has a dual polarity. The energy of Pluto aptly describes the principle resulting from Divine will's experience through the creation, but until fairly recently this emanative aspect was attributed to a hypothetical planet called Vulcan. It doesn't matter what label you give to a symbol that represents a particular aspect, as long as the quality or principle itself is understood. In 1977, a minor planet was discovered whose orbit lies for the most part between Saturn and Uranus, which would appropriately place it upon the middle pillar of the Tree and in the space formerly assigned to Vulcan. This planet, Chiron, is known as the wounded healer. Its healing is the pure and balanced will of God as it goes forth into the world; this will becomes wounded when its expression through man results in an impure and unbalanced world. The symbol for Chiron is the centaur, a creature that has the body and limbs of a horse and

65

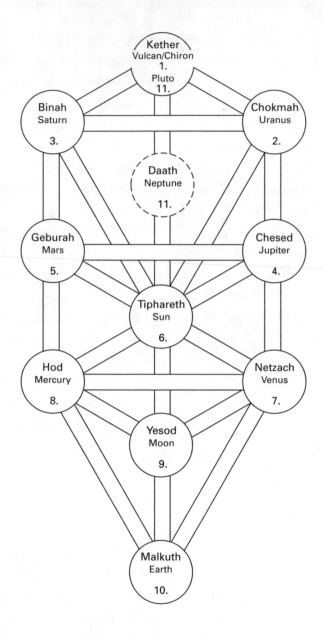

FIGURE 8.1. THE PRINCIPLES OF DIVINE EXPRESSION
SYMBOLIZED BY PLANETARY ENERGIES

the torso, arms, and head of a human. Here in this symbol is represented the journey of man from the powerful instinctual level to the development of his humanity. The mythological story of Chiron, when interpreted on the esoteric level, places this aspect on Kether of the Tree.

Note that the moon, representing Yesod, is not a planet but a satellite of the planet Earth. Many feel that this also is a temporary position, resulting from man's attachment to his past, and that one day a new planet will be discovered that will more aptly describe the freedom of man's response to his soul. And, although we look at the Tree as a glyph or diagram, we must remember that it is an archetypal symbol; as such, it has been endowed with a life of its own, a very powerful and empowering life.

67

A principle is defined as the basic or essential element determining intrinsic nature; also, a basic source. As stated previously, the Sephiroth represent Divine principles that constitute what we might term "the body of God." Created in the image of God, man—an expressive/creative being expresses those same principles through his creativity. We can never describe these principles as they relate to Divinity, but we can describe them as they relate to man, for they are the principles assigned to those planets that represent the Sephiroth.

A principle expresses itself into a quality, a characteristic most compatible with its expression. We could say that the quality is the ideal form or containment for the force of the principle. If man expresses a principle properly, the resultant quality will be evident. However, that quality can further be expressed in either a positive or negative manner. Consider, for example, the principle of electricity, which we could say is a principle of force.

Its quality could be said to be enlivenment, which could be used to either cure or kill. This is a rather rudimentary example, but it gives an idea of how the principle and quality are neither good nor bad; it is their application that can be defined as such.

The list on page 69 shows each Sephirah's planetary representation, principle, quality, positive expression, and negative expression. Since pure Divine will is emanated from Kether, we can define its principle and quality, but it is nearly impossible to define positive or negative expressions as they apply to transcendence. We can define only those aspects as they are transformed down to man's levels of duality.

In regard to Kabalistic healing, we are concerned with the results of the positive and negative expressions, these results being the most evident in life. Like the expressions, the results can be either positive or negative. The positive results exhibit themselves in what we call virtues, bringing balance and harmony into the life experience, while the negative results, called vices, produce imbalance, disharmony, and disease.

We align these results in accordance with the planetary energies, this time defining their positive and negative aspects. Each Sephirah on the Tree of Life is assigned a virtue and a vice. These can be further expanded upon by those aspects related to the Sephiroth's planetary representations.

The terms in bold are the traditional virtues and vices of the Sephiroth, while the other descriptions of the planetary forces as they relate to the Sephiroth clarify the traits and characteristics that evidence themselves through the lives of individuals. These are just a few descriptions; many more can be found in a good book on astrology, which should further identify the

SEPHIRAH	PLANET	PRINCIPLE	QUALITY	POSITIVE EXPRESSION	NEGATIVE EXPRESSION
1. Kether	Chiron	Emanation	Wisdom	Sublimation	Repression
2. Chokmah	Uranus	Transformation	Originality	Inventiveness	Deviance
3. Binah	Saturn	Limitation	Restraint	Discipline	Crystallization
4. Chesed	Jupiter	Expansion	Foresight	Optimism	Extravagance
5. Geburah	Mars	Projection	Forcefulness	Vigor	Aggression
6. Tiphareth	Sun	Power	Individuality	Magnanimity	Egotism
7. Netzach	Venus	Attraction	Beauty	Grace	Sensuality
8. Hod	Mercury	Communication	Intelligence	Discernment	Variability
9. Yesod	Moon	Response	Sensitivity	Empathy	Moodiness
10. Malkuth	Earth	Embodiment	Practicality	Common sense	Materialism
11. Daath	Neptune	Transcendence	Vision	Idealism	Escapism
12. Kether	Pluto	Resurrection	Determination	Resoluteness	Coercion

SEPHIRAH	PLANET	VIRTUE	VICE
1. Kether	Chiron	**attainment**	**atheism**
2. Chokmah	Uranus	**devotion,** altruism, inventiveness, perceptiveness, spontaneity	**misused power,** rebelliousness, irresponsibility, unpredictability, eccentricity, radicalism
3. Binah	Saturn	**silence,** patience, restraint, self-discipline, conservatism, stability	**avarice,** greed, secrecy pessimism, rigidity, vengeance
4. Chesed	Jupiter	**obedience,** enthusiasm, optimism, benevolence, tolerance, idealism	**waste, gluttony, tyranny,** bigotry, extravagance, gullibility, laziness, fanaticism
5. Geburah	Mars	**energy, courage,** power, endurance, stamina, activity, heroism	**cruelty, destruction,** aggressiveness, impulsiveness, selfishness, dominance, violence
6. Tiphareth	Sun	**devotion to the Great Work,** creativity, vitality, leadership, confidence, generosity	**pride,** pomposity, conceit, contemptuousness, willfulness, bluntness

#		Positive	Negative
7. Netzach	Venus	**selflessness,** cooperativity, refinement, consideration, sociability, appreciation	**lust, misused sex,** promiscuity, indifference, superficiality, temperamentalness, self-indulgence, impracticality
8. Hod	Mercury	**truthfulness,** alertness, versatility, dexterity, agility, expressiveness	**falsehood, dishonesty, criticism,** skepticism, restlessness, indecisiveness, criticalness, worry
9. Yesod	Moon	**independence,** receptivity, empathy, flexibility, protectiveness, patience, love	**idleness,** touchiness, moodiness, insensitivity, inconsistency, smothering
10. Malkuth	Earth	**diagnosis, discrimination,** productivity, thoroughness, reliability, perseverance, practicality	**inertia, avarice,** stubbornness, materialism, selfishness, possessiveness, laziness
11. Daath	Neptune	**detachment,** vision, spiritual wisdom, inspiration, universal love, responsiveness	**corruption, doubt, cowardice,** fear, escapism, confusion, attachment, insecurity
12. Kether	Pluto	**attainment,** transformation, illumination, regeneration, freedom, spirituality	**atheism,** lawlessness, destruction, combat, obsessiveness, recklessness

principles of Divinity as they are expressed by man. Knowledge of these virtues and vices is essential for the professional in Kabalistic healing, for just as a physician is thoroughly acquainted with the physical body, the Kabalistic healer must be acquainted with the body called "man."

Simpler techniques for Kabalistic healing that can be used by those who are not acquainted with the Tree, as well as by those who know the Tree but have not integrated the highest level of Kabalistic healing, will be presented later in this book. Remember that the Tree is a powerful archetype and that simply acknowledging it instigates a response within the unconscious mind. In many of his writings, Carl Jung emphasized that the one who speaks in primordial images (archetypal symbols) has the voice of a thousand trumpets. These images elevate the meaning of the symbol from the individual and transitory level into the eternal. Primordial symbols are archetypes; as such, the Tree of Life reflects to man the reality of existence.

Think of the principles of the Tree as medications. Aspirin can be purchased to relieve a headache, but if the headache is caused by a brain tumor, then a specialist must be consulted. That specialist must have a thorough knowledge of not only the problem but also the possible remedies used to correct it. It is much the same with Kabalistic healing: some distortions require simple applications of energy and only a basic knowledge of remedies, while others demand the services of one who has become proficient in that field.

9

The Expression
of Man
Through Mankind

U p to now, we have investigated man's world—the World of
Yetzirah—and mankind's world, the World of Assiah. Now
we will see how man expresses through mankind. This can best
be explained by the overlaying of these two Worlds shown in figure 9.1. Interaction between Worlds occurs as the lower half of
one World expresses itself into the upper half of the next lower
World. This direction from a higher to lower authority results in
what we call a "hierarchical" universe, one in which something
lower responds to that which is higher. In Genesis, God gave
man dominion over every creeping thing upon the earth; thus
man has dominion over those kingdoms of lower consciousness.

Figure 9.1 depicts the interaction between man and
mankind. The lower half of the World of Yetzirah, man's creative
world, overlays and directly interacts with the upper half of the

World of Assiah, the formative world. This interaction takes place within the world of mankind. The pure will or intent of the Divine within man extends from its source in Kether of Yetzirah through all levels, empowering each with the mandate to exist, and finally reaches its culmination in the physical body of mankind. Each level of this intent takes upon itself a consciousness or knowing relative to that level. Of course, the World of Yetzirah has an interaction with the next higher World of Briah, as does the World of Briah with the World of Atziluth, but for the purpose of understanding Kabalistic healing, it is the Worlds of Yetzirah and Assiah with which we must be concerned. Suffice it to say that the Divine will within man, originating in Kether, has already descended through two higher Worlds.

In figure 9.1, where the Trees overlap, the functions relative to the higher World are printed in the upper half of the Sephiroth; those relating to the lower World are printed in the lower half. In its evolution man's consciousness has already ascended through the World of Assiah, the stages of infancy and childhood. At present, consciousness is growing within the lower half of the World of Yetzirah, the half that is man's creative world. Placing the collective consciousness of man upon the Yetziratic Tree, it extends from Yesod to Tiphareth. In actuality and in keeping pace with universal evolution, all of mankind should be in consciousness above the path that joins Netzach and Hod of Yetzirah.

Ascending the Tree, the first point of interaction is found in Tiphareth of Assiah, the brain and central nervous system, as it is overlaid by Malkuth of Yetzirah, the conscious mind. This overleaving demonstrates that the brain is a tool for the functioning of that mind. Because the conscious mind is the recipient of all of the higher influences within its World, its efficiency

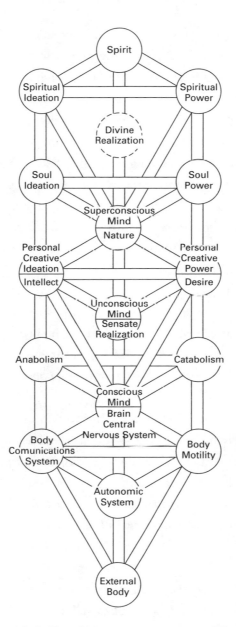

75

FIGURE 9.1. THE INTERACTION OF THE WORLDS
OF MAN AND MANKIND

is determined by the evolutionary status of consciousness. A conscious mind unable to receive any higher influence due to its limitations would influence the brain in much the same manner as primitive man's did. The conscious mind expresses its will/intent into the external world and is vitally important to the functioning of mankind in that world. The senses determine what the brain perceives; then the mind reasons about what the brain determines from its perception. Therefore, the brain directs the physical body in its activity or movement. Along with being utilized by the conscious mind from the next higher World, the physical body is also influenced by the higher level within its own World, which contains the senses as well as the principles of desire and intellect.

76

The next higher overlaying principles are those of Daath of Assiah, sensate realization, overlaid by the principle of Yesod of Yetzirah, the unconscious mind. Unconscious reactions are usually based on feelings that form the unconscious's means of expression.

The principles of force and form used on both levels by these overlaying aspects of will also overlay each other: Chokmah of Assiah (desire) and Binah of Assiah (intellect) are overlaid by Netzach of Yetzirah (personal creative power) and Hod of Yetzirah (personal creative ideation). Man's growth, beginning in the very primitive stage, was based on his instinctual nature—his "fight or flight" response. He slowly developed the principles of intellect and desire/motivation, which, like the brain, are tools essential for the functioning of mankind and vital for the growth of man's consciousness. However, these are principles that should be used by man, not identified with man.

Intellect and desire/motivation are the highest principles in the World of Assiah, and they continue to be empowered and refined as man's consciousness grows. Sensate realization depends upon those principles, since they are the determinants through which life is experienced.

Mankind's intellect, Binah of Assiah, and desire/motivation, Chokmah of Assiah, are overlaid by man's creative ideation, Hod of Yetzirah, and creative power, Netzach of Yetzirah. These overlaying principles are the only ones on the side pillars of the Tree that directly relate to the interaction between man and mankind. Being of higher frequencies, man's creative ideation and power should direct those principles of intellect and desire/motivation of the next lower world. The creative functions of man should direct the sensate functions of mankind. However, since man's unconscious mind has been programmed to believe that it is the external world, its powerful will is governed by the sensate will of the lower world.

Man identifies with his external existence. He establishes that identity by his titles, his vocation, his possessions, and the attributes by which others define him. With the power of the statement "I am," man identifies himself with the vehicle through which he experiences life. And if those aspects with which he identifies are in some way taken from him, he is lost. All of the above-mentioned aspects can define existence, but they should not define man. Man even identifies with the senses. How often we hear "I am happy" or "I am sad," both of which can be translated as "I identify myself as a sensate expression." This identification only reinforces the attachment of the unconscious mind to sensate realization. Man has become a being composed of sensate

77

principles that govern his creative ability, which is why distortion, chaos, and disease run rampant in our world.

When one says "I am tired," this conscious statement directs the will of the unconscious to create tiredness. When one says "I am ill," the unconscious creates illness. In truth, man *feels* tired; he *feels* ill. He feels it because it is present in his vehicle, the body, and his sensate realization is reporting that condition to him so that he may take creative action for correcting the distortion, whatever it may be.

What has happened? Why does man not only identify with his senses and external world but is, in a sense, addicted to them? In the beginning, it was a natural part of the growth process, just as a child learns about his world through games and role-playing, an important part of the growing-up process. Through such experiences and his interaction with other children in these processes, the child prepares himself for his adult status, wherein he expresses himself into the "real world" that his childhood experiences prepared him for. As the child gradually matures he releases those play experiences and, in fact, desires more and more to experience as an adult. Toy cars are abandoned for a real automobile; however, with the acquisition of an automobile comes the responsibility of driving one. Toy car crashes affect little around them, while automobile crashes affect the lives and well-being of others. As a child, one has to identify as a child; but in order to function properly as an adult in the world, one must identify as an adult. In both childhood and adulthood, one must be able to function in accord with his status.

Man's evolution in consciousness took him from instinctual to intellectual man, the height of the world of mankind.

Here, man became a sort of god within the world of mankind. Collectively, man should be reaching the level of superconscious mind or will, Tiphareth of Yetzirah, and the development of intuition relating to that status. Intuition does not mean that some higher or Divine guidance directs man in his every activity. Instead, man draws upon his inner teaching ("in-tuition") to live his life as a spiritual adult, much like the child who, upon reaching maturity, draws upon his past educational process of life in order to express his adulthood.

As long as man's psyche believes itself to be a sensate being whose principles of intellect and desire define his existence, rather than enable him to express freely within it, he simply re-creates his evolutionary life as a child who long ago should have grown beyond that state of existence. This is verified by the "I need" and "I want" criteria of man's present world. Childlike qualities of greed, possessiveness, anger, hostility, self-centeredness, fear, and so on rule the greater part of man's world. This is reflected into every aspect of life, as well as into the distortion and disease within mankind that reflect these higher distorted principles.

The Exodus story of the Israelites' bondage in Egypt symbolizes man's bondage to physical existence; the plagues relate to the misuse of man's Divine principles, a misuse resulting in ever more intense distortions in the world. Looking at the Worlds of Mankind and Man, we can attribute the halves of those Worlds to the growth of man's consciousness. The lower half of Assiah, the realm of the physical body, relates to the infancy stage, where, like an infant, man adapted to the vehicle he would use during the growth of his consciousness. He was "born" instinctual, and during his infancy began to develop his intellectual/desire nature.

79

As this nature became viable the infant grew into childhood, continuing his development and education through the upper half of the World of Assiah. Studying ancient history, we find that the desire nature, as well as intellect, were highly developed some 3,000 years ago, with desire (force) directing the intellect (form). What man desired required an intellect to acquire.

As the power or strength of consciousness continued to increase, due to its empowerment by Universal nature, man's creative ability developed. This is much like the body of a child, which gains strength simply by virtue of its growth. A child of five is able to lift a greater weight than a child of one. As stated previously, the power of will increases as a result of Universal nature. Being dual in nature, the power of will within man can either promote growth or crystallize it; thus man was invested even more greatly in those structures that his potential indicated he was ready to move beyond. As intellect and desire were strengthened, man's creative ability, the strength of will of the unconscious, was also empowered; he began to create existence based on intellect and desire, rather than merely using these principles. Thus creative ideation and creative power were, and continue to be, dominated by the sensate principles of intellect and desire. In a sense, mankind, the vehicle, operates or drives man in the direction and manner of the vehicle's choosing, rather than in the direction that is appropriate for man. The upper half of Assiah is the formative world; that is to say, it forms the substance of the material world in accordance with the realization that directs it. This realization, Daath of Assiah, should be governed by the unconscious mind's will, as it responds to the adult will of man, Tiphareth of Yetzirah. However, because unconscious will identifies with sensate realization and its world, it cannot respond to the higher influence of Tiphareth, also known as the superconscious, soul, or Self. Tiphareth represents the status of a mature will, while Malkuth is the infant and Yesod is the child. Simply said, man is endeavoring to live the life of an adult with a child's consciousness and has become, like a thirty-year-old with the mind of a five-year-old, dangerous to himself and his world.

Tiphareth of Yetzirah overlays Kether of Assiah, the will of nature in that World. As the center of beauty, balance, and harmony, whatever Tiphareth would have dominion over should reflect these qualities. But in order to achieve this level of growth, man must detach from his childhood, bringing the development of that period of growth into an adult status wherein life could be experienced without the extremes of disease and distortion. The journey to that adult status becomes more difficult as man resists it.

81

Breaking the identification with and, indeed, the addiction to the sensate world of mankind requires much the same effort that is required to break any addiction. The withdrawal symptoms are similar. The process requires understanding, determination, and most important, supportive guidance on whatever level it is needed: physical, emotional, and/or creative. Physicians furnish such support on the physical level, therapists and psychologists on the emotional level, and Kabalistic healers on the creative, or soul, level. The more detachment the Kabalistic healer achieves from the sensate world of mankind, and the more able he is to reach the will of the soul, or superconscious, the more effective his healing will be. Therefore, self-development becomes primary to

Kabalistic healing, and this involves a transformational process such as that found in the Kabalah itself.

To summarize, the growth of man's consciousness is contained in the Worlds of Assiah and Yetzirah, from its establishment of familiarity with the kingdom through which it becomes viable—the kingdom of mankind—to the realization and understanding of the reality of its existence. The realms that relate to mankind are those of Assiah—the active, or physical, and the formative or sensate worlds; those that relate to man are the creative and the spiritual, or Divine, worlds contained in Yetzirah. Man and mankind constitute a singular totality; one could not exist without the other. Consciousness develops through the experiences of man/mankind, while the two terms, *man* and *mankind,* can be used to connote the spiritual or evolutionary age of consciousness, personally and collectively. In accordance with the evolutionary plan for the family of man, consciousness should have evolved through the physical and formative stages of growth—these being related to the infancy and childhood stages—and should be assuming the adult status. But by lagging behind in the life educational process, consciousness has attained the power of adulthood but retained the knowledge of a child; thus, disharmony continually increases within the world of mankind. Just as we interrelate with each other through definition of form, we must now begin to realize ourselves as mind-beings who experience through that form. It is still necessary to define it, but we should not identify with it.

In looking at the diagram of the overlaying Trees depicting the man/mankind totality, you can see that the distortion has occurred in the transition of consciousness from childhood to maturity, as man, for whatever reason, refused to assume the higher education and responsibility needed to encompass his adult expression. Childhood concepts instilled in the unconscious mind must be reformed and/or corrected, so that man can complete the "individuation of the Self," as Jung terms it. Man does indeed have dominion over his world, but should exercise this dominion only with a level of consciousness, or knowing, that works for the common good of all. The process of Kabalah goes far deeper than this brief description, but for the purpose of understanding Kabalistic healing this will be sufficient.

Relating to everything in existence, the Tree of Life can be used to understand this nature of man/mankind, just as a diagram of the anatomy of mankind enables the physician to practice medicine. The diagram itself does nothing, but the knowledge and application of what it portrays empowers the physician. Kabalistic healers can be considered "soul physicians," and just like those who study medicine, they require the development that enables their practice.

83

10

Pain

In the previous chapters we discussed the life-will of Divinity as it develops principles of itself, and of its dual expressions of force and form through the worlds and levels of man/mankind. Existing within four levels (spiritual, creative, formative or astral, and physical), consciousness coalesces a form viable upon each of those levels. Thus within the physical bodies of mankind, there are also contained what we could term emotional/intellectual— or astral—bodies, creative bodies, and spiritual bodies. A distortion in the application of any of the Divine principles within any or all of these bodies results in the symptom of that distortion, which is called pain. There is physical pain, emotional/intellectual pain, creative pain, and spiritual pain.

There is probably no one in the world who has not experienced pain, since it is a normal part of the growth process.

Mankind reacts to pain in many ways: he fights it, he becomes enraged at it, he succumbs to it in self-pity, he talks about it, but most of all, he fails to understand it. The word *pain* is derived from the same Latin word as the word *punish,* which enhances the fact that it is something "bad." We view pain as something to be avoided at all costs, instead of something to be investigated other than for the purpose of relieving it.

Pain fulfills the law of action and reaction (for every action there is an equal and opposite reaction) upon the levels in which duality exists. Here it is the opposite of pleasure. Pain produces feelings of sadness, sorrow, anger, frustration, and despair, while pleasure produces feelings of elation, happiness, and joy. Although seemingly at opposite ends of the spectrum, these feelings are actually the same energies; the sensations they produce are defined by the result of their application. What must be understood is that pain is no more an enemy than pleasure, and each can either serve or deter man in the growth process of his life experience.

From the beginning of time, man has looked to external causes for the pain he has endured. At first man believed he was being punished by the nature gods; then it was a singular God who inflicted punishment for a "sin" that man committed but often could not even understand. Thus the concept of God became associated with cruelty and unjustness. Even as man reaches the understanding that as the creator of his reality he is also the creator of his pain, he still most often feels he has done something wrong that has justified the pain. Pain becomes an enemy, rather than a friend that by its very existence is endeavoring to tell man that disharmony exists on some level. Rather than fight the pain, man should endeavor to correct the dishar-mony, which would make the pain disappear.

Sometimes pain may be a punishment, but there are many other reasons for its existence. Often it is an indication of what must be gained or acquired in the present cycle of life. If an individual has not learned to read, he incurs emotional/intellectual pain as he tries to live in an adult world, where the ability to read is of prime importance. In our life journey, pain often indicates which Divine principles must be integrated or focused on. Pain is an important motivator in the journey of life. Remember that the beingness of man, that Divine spark created in the image of its Creator, clothed itself in forms relative to each level of its descent into the world, these levels decreasing in vibratory fre-quency until the physical world of matter was reached. Even though that initial spark reflects its pure Divine source, it cannot influence the denser bodies until they reach a degree of perfec-tion or balance that enables them to comply with pure Divine will. This state is that of spiritual maturity, the adulthood status represented by Tiphareth of Yetzirah upon the Tree of Life.

The application of pain in an individual life span serves to convey to man the knowledge of law or truth, beginning at the lowest level and continuing to each succeeding level of growth achieved by consciousness. Much like an infant, primi-tive man first had to learn what he was not and develop a sense of himself separate from his surroundings. Some things with which he interacted caused pain; others produced pleasure. Mankind began to want pleasurable experiences and to avoid those that caused pain, but without the pain, he would not have learned to avoid them. Thus he came to learn the laws that apply to physical living, and he learned that breaking these laws, either deliberately or inadvertently, leads to pain. He also learned that what was pleasurable and even desirable could also produce pain when used inappropriately. Through this process man gained experience and accumulated knowledge, which enabled him to regulate his desires through pain. Man now had the ability to guide and educate his lower nature through his developing intellect and desire. Without pain, man would have never grown beyond that primitive stage.

This period was to man's evolutionary life what infancy is to an individual life span. A child often suffers many bumps and bruises as he discovers his external world. Learning to crawl and then walk, he crashes into solid objects, or he stumbles and falls. Because a child's memory span is very short, he forgets the pain in his desire for mobility, and although he cries when he feels the pain again, it is soon forgotten in that desire. As a child matures, his bones become more brittle; the kind of fall from which a child arises very quickly can be dangerous to an adult. Similarly, as man grows in awareness, he suffers greater damage to the foundational structure of his consciousness if he "falls," or breaks the laws that his experience has made him aware of.

On the next higher intellectual/emotional level, pain is used for the gradual dissipation of desire. Desire and self-gratification were necessary means for man to learn about his external world, but in order to achieve adult status man must learn that he is not his desires. Desire is not an inappropriate feeling, but it must be used by man rather than control him, as is so often the case in today's society. Man still must gain knowledge through experience within the external world, but if the desire for an object remains, then the knowledge integrated cannot become a part of his soul or adult consciousness.

At first, as every desire is gratified, the pleasure derived from it becomes more intense, leading one to seek that gratification again and again, without realizing that upon the sensate level there is no satiation point. Also, what one desires is transitory and temporary, and the intervals in which one cannot have the object of his pleasure are painful. Pleasure itself is transitory and temporary. Thus when the objects of man's pleasure are inevitably removed from him, even greater pain is inflicted. Since desire is a fundamental aspect of man's personality, when he leaves the physical body in death the desire still remains, even though the object of that desire is no longer in his plane of existence.

Because man identifies with his external world and its physical and sensate realms, the physical and intellectual/emotional bodies encounter the greatest experiences with pain. Pain results from this misidentification and is a symptom of a distortion or disease, either emotional or physical. Emotional distortions, if allowed to persist, will eventually manifest within the physical vehicle as disease.

Pain also serves to strengthen consciousness; this strength, which relates to the creative body, is an aspect of spiritual maturity. It is neither physical nor emotional strength, but what we might call strength of character. Spiritually, it has been called faith. Faith relates to the maturation process of man by the establishment of the surety or certainty of his existence, which upon the next lower level is translated into self-worth, and upon the next, confidence. The highest aspect is a state of being, which on the levels below it is a state of knowing and finally a state of doing.

As the highest state, being empowers those lower levels. Through the experiences of everyday life and its stress, strife, and trials, man comes not only to know who he is but to become who he is. One rarely seeks to understand himself or his life until he is beset by pain. Man's inherent nature is to create, and that creativity relates to the life experience. If life were comfortable, man would not be willing to change it, nor would he exercise his creativity without being forced to do so. Change is the only constant in the universe, and man's change reflects his growth.

The final level of pain relates to the spiritual body and is difficult to define, since it manifests as an emptiness or inner hunger that cannot be satiated by anything external. When man experiences this pain, he first identifies it as something that is "missing" from the other levels of his existence, but then finds that nothing from those levels can appease the pain. It is the pain of the "call," the beckoning impact of Divine Spirit that draws man toward the reality of his existence. That reality exists with man's being, not in the "real" world of mankind. Mankind's real and tangible world exists for the purpose of man's experiential growth into the reality of man's world. When that occurs, mankind's world will reflect the beauty and harmony of the world of reality, and pain will diminish.

Pain's impact is present upon the bodies within which Divine life becomes clothed, but it is not part of the essential nature of that Divine life. In the evolutionary life of man, pain is at first an enemy, but soon man comes to realize that pain is a friend that indicates where a distortion or weakness exists. Then he can begin to focus his efforts on the correction of the distortion. To focus attention or energy on the pain itself only strengthens it and increases its intensity as a symptom. It also detracts energy that could be directed to correcting the distortion. Pain is not the problem, but it indicates the problem. Pain protects man's body. If one places his hand into a fire, the resultant pain indicates that damage can result from such an action. The conscious memory of the pain prevents man from repeating the incident. The unconscious memory of emotional pain prevents one from entering into a situation similar to that which caused the pain; however, memory does not bring the same degree of pain that was experienced in the original incident. The greater the passage of time, the less the unconscious "recalls" pain. Therefore, if one repeats the situation, he will again incur the symptomatic pain until the lesson the experience was designed to teach is learned. It is not the pain the unconscious remembers, but the reactions to the experience in which pain was incurred. Oftentimes, merely a key-in to that experience will produce a reaction, and similar pain will result with no apparent external reason. A key-in is something within a present situation which is similar to something in a past situation in which pain was encountered. For instance, seeing a dog might produce a reaction to it based upon a previous incident in which one was bitten by a dog. Much like a certain key on a computer brings up a whole program, there are keys in life which elicit a reactive program based upon certain past experiences. Pain within the emotional body most often translates into pain within the physical body, and so mankind experiences a myriad of aches and pains that are often totally unrelated to his actual physical actions.

As a creator, what man thinks and speaks is often responsible for the distortion that causes the symptom of pain. For instance, if one believes he is carrying too great a burden, the unconscious translates this literally into the physical body as a distortion of the pattern for the skeleton. Back pain ensues, and the individual wonders what he has done to injure it. If he can move beyond this idea, reach the understanding that his thoughts created the problem, and correct the concept held in his thoughts, then often the pain will disappear instantly. The pain has done its job, for it has drawn attention to an emotional/intellectual distortion. However, if the thought has been held for a long time and involves relationships between one individual and another, then the relieving of the back pain becomes more complex, necessitating help and guidance upon the physical, emotional, and, often, creative levels. It is important to remember that your creative ability uses the patterns of your unconscious/conscious belief system to establish physical form.

92

Pain is a symptom of distortion, not the cause of it. Its purpose is to draw attention to what either needs to be corrected or needs to be integrated. Focusing on the pain only increases its intensity, as does ignoring the distortion to which the pain is attempting to draw your attention. One takes steps to relieve the pain as far as necessity demands, but at the same time one must turn his attention to the problem it indicates. Pain is a natural process of growth, for until man detaches from his identification with the external world, pain is the motivator for developing those principles that complete his wholeness. With the development of that wholeness is established a world of beauty, balance, and harmony, wherein man continues to evolve through his own efforts, rather than under the sway of the forces that mandate his existence.

11

Disease

In the previous chapter, pain was shown to be a symptom of disease; thus it is now important to understand just what disease is. The word *disease* is comprised of two parts: *dis,* meaning "apart" or "opposite of," and *ease,* meaning "a state of being comfortable" or "freedom from pain or discomfort." Therefore, disease the "opposite of comfort"—is the establishment of disharmony or imbalance within mankind's experience. We can find disease within the physical, emotional, and creative levels of being. Why does this occur? Simply, disease is a reflection of the distortion of Divine life-will as it expresses through inappropriate concepts held by man relative to the stage of his evolutionary growth. It is a lack of harmony between life-will and its physical expression. Disease does not always result from something that man has done wrong, but can be a valuable learning experience designed to enhance both one's personal growth pattern and the collective pattern of all mankind.

We must also take into account that disease exists not just within the kingdom of mankind, but in the lower kingdoms as well; namely, the mineral, plant, and animal kingdoms. Imbalance may occur within these kingdoms as a result of their growth processes, but we must also take into consideration that man's dominion over these kingdoms includes the projection of his disharmony upon them. Disease is a fact in nature. And just as pain is a symptom of disease, disease itself is a symptom of imbalance on some level. Regardless of the level upon which an imbalance occurs, it will eventually manifest itself within the physical form of the body. Even what we call emotional disease leads to physical debilitation.

We can define three aspects of disease in an ever-widening spectrum. The first aspect relates to man's projection into manifestation—what we call life experience—which we are continually in the process of learning about. The second aspect relates to mankind as a whole; that is, the collective experience or collective consciousness of mankind, which we are just beginning to understand. Remember that mankind comprises the totality of one Divine life, in which each fragment or cell contains the properties of its Source, much like the drop of ocean water contains all the properties of the body of water from which it was derived. The third aspect, of which we know little, relates to planetary life, or the totality of man in its relationship to the cosmos.

Disease, or disharmony, is also governed by the law of cause and effect, also known as *karma*. Karma is frequently portrayed as some sort of payback or punishment, but this is not necessarily the case. Karma is the product of three factors relative to the three aspects of disease. The first factor relates to man's personality—his past as well as what he is presently capable of integrating. The word *karma* comes from a Sanskrit word meaning "action." Action can be classified as either good or bad, but all action contributes to growth. The second factor of karma relates to the totality of mankind, which each person inherits as his part of the responsibility for the totality. The third factor, man shares with all the natural forms within all kingdoms, and thus relates to planetary life, about which little is understood at this time.

In earlier chapters it was shown that individual and collective consciousness, upon whatever level they are centered, create existence. If the concepts or patterns held by consciousness are inappropriate for any reason, then distortion results. That distortion, as stated previously, will show itself within the life experience of mankind. Thus for healing, or establishment of "ease," to occur, one must understand what has created the distortion. For harmony to exist within the totality of mankind, each individual must first establish it within himself. And therein lies karma. Each individual has an innate urge to establish harmony, but may instead create one imbalance in an ineffectual attempt to correct another.

Just as with pain, man views disease in anger, frustration, and fear, rather than endeavoring to understand what the symptom of disease indicates. It is important to remember that disease always promotes liberation and destroys crystallization. It is designed to promote the integration of a quality or attribute, and once that quality or attribute is acquired, a cure is possible. Disease may also be the process consciousness uses to withdraw from its current habitation. This withdrawal can be quick and unexpected, or extended over a long period of time.

Since man, for the most part, can relate only to what he sees and feels, it is necessary for undesirable subjective conditions to become externalized, so that they can then be known, dealt with, and eliminated. Sometimes this elimination brings death to the physical vehicle, whereupon consciousness is liberated to establish a new vehicle that is free from the eliminated condition. If certain undesirable conditions persist from lifetime to lifetime, they will continue to worsen. Ignoring the symptoms of disease only causes it to worsen, just as ignoring the pain of an aching tooth does not correct the problem. One can take a painkiller to relieve the pain of an aching tooth, but the problem only continues, often until it becomes necessary to remove the tooth.

How consciousness impacts the physical body can be understood by studying the overlaying Trees of man and mankind. The lower half of man's Tree, Yetzirah—the realm of consciousness—overlays the upper half of mankind's Tree, Assiah—the formative realm of particles, waves, atoms, and molecules. This is the world of mankind over which man was given dominion, a dominion that has become stronger as man has grown toward spiritual maturity. Man has become a greatly empowered creator, but because of his identification/attachment with the external world, he creates with concepts more appropriate for his spiritual childhood than for his maturity. Remember that the body of mankind is created from the formative realm. Inappropriate patterns create a distorted vehicle, and the resulting disease endeavors to indicate and pinpoint those inappropriate patterns so they can be corrected.

Man's creative power and creative ideation overlay the dual aspects of desire and intellect of mankind and are at present dominated by them; thus, as many texts state, man's thinking and feeling, if used inappropriately, create disease.

As stated earlier, disease can be individual, collective, or universal. An example of collective distortion is indicated in the existence of viruses and bacteria. One's own immunity determines his reaction to these. There is a direct correlation between the heart chakra, its corresponding endocrine gland—the thymus—and the establishment of immunity. By the time an individual is about fourteen years old, the immunity pattern is established and the thymus atrophies. Additional or increased immunity must then come forth from the heart center, represented by Tiphareth upon the Tree. Through the virtue of that Sephirah, devotion to the Great Work, the heart chakra is stimulated, thereby increasing immunity within the physical body. Devotion to the Great Work simply means following one's own life pattern as it fulfills its part within the total pattern for all mankind. This devotion requires the integration of the principles through which it expresses, Hod and Netzach, whose virtues are truth and selflessness, respectively. The lack of integration of these two virtues is responsible for many of the illnesses seen in the world today. Truth relates to the realization of one's individualism, not what someone else tells him he is nor what his feelings define him as. Selflessness relates to life expression that serves all mankind, not just the personal self. To develop selflessness, one must detach from the evolutionary childhood self and integrate with the evolutionary mature Self. This is the mature Self as defined by Jung: superconsciousness, also called the soul. Much of mankind does not consciously acknowledge selflessness, which is necessary for expression as a spiritual adult.

Because of this, we see a great influx of immunity-related diseases, not only in mankind but in the lower kingdoms as well.

One of the most common diseases running rampant in mankind is influenza, of which there are innumerable types and degrees of severity. When we break down the symptoms of influenza into its components, we see a clear picture of what is occurring within mankind's growth process at this time. It shows mankind's resistance to growth, as well as a representation of what occurs in the growth process. The symptoms are very symbolic and include diarrhea, a purging of that which one has previously assimilated; vomiting, a purging of that which is not fit to be assimilated; aches and pains, growing pains, and/or resistance to growth; congestion, a blockage to the truth of the reality of one's existence; and fever, an indication of an influx of life-will serving as an impetus to promote growth. Since immunity to disease relates to the Tiphareth—the heart center of consciousness—then a lowered resistance to this disease would indicate that one has not integrated the Tiphareth level of consciousness to the degree one is capable of and that one is probably invested in the self—the personal self, with a lowercase *s*. It is the personal self that has invested its childlike nature in the negative application of the principles of force and form, Netzach and Hod, principles used by the varying levels of the growth of consciousness.

The presence of a disease usually draws even more attention to the self, as one becomes vested in self-pity, despair, and frustration, along with fear about his mortality. The illness then intensifies, endeavoring to show that one's focus is misdirected, whereupon the individual becomes even more greatly invested in self. Sometimes, the only way to break this vicious cycle is for consciousness to withdraw from the physical body, a withdrawal known as death. There may come a time when the physical vehicle cannot tolerate any further distortion of the pattern appropriate for it and death is the only way a new vehicle can be acquired. This does not cure the affliction, for the new vehicle will either be born containing a distortion (disease) or will have a predisposition to it.

Kabalistic healing identifies three major areas that are affected by disease, which become the foundation upon which each physical manifestation is created. These areas are will or power, affecting respiration; equality of rhythm, affecting the heart, circulatory system, and nervous system; and activity or foundation, affecting assimilation and elimination. These also represent the creative, emotional/intellectual, and physical levels as they express through the physical body. While all three of these levels are prominent in our world, the most greatly affected is the emotional/intellectual level, in which man is immersed in consciousness. Here, the imbalance is seen in the many diseases of the heart, circulatory system, and especially of the nervous system that are common in our world. The sale of antidepressants and mood elevators is at an all-time high.

What we term disease and most often see as an alien, external enemy is actually the physical manifestation of our own personal and collective belief systems. Man creates the distortions, and thus he can "uncreate" them by attaining that which the distortion indicates is lacking or needs to be integrated within the being called man. Mankind ("like a man") reflects this distortion as disease within the body. While temporary cures may

99

alleviate the body's affliction, the distortion still remains within man—its creator—and until it is corrected, a permanent cure cannot take place. Even though permanent cures seem to occur, these usually are relative to one life cycle, unless the individual has reached that place in his growth cycle where a permanent cure is possible.

It is also important to understand that an individual who appears to be in good health is not necessarily higher in spiritual awareness than an individual who has many afflictions. Certainly, the attainment of a higher awareness does bring balance and thus good health to the body, but just as in the educational process of life, there are school sessions and there are vacations. A vacation in this case does not indicate a time for nongrowth, but rather gives the individual a time to demonstrate what has been gained in previous educational sessions. There are readjustments made within every cycle, and even when a healthy individual is in a time of rest, so to speak, a new cycle may loom on the horizon. It is important to view life as an ongoing process in which what is gained in each cycle will be demonstrated in the next.

12

Understanding
Disease

The previous chapter defined disease as a state of "dis-ease, the opposite of freedom from pain or discomfort," resulting in distortion or imbalance within any of those levels that make up mankind. Correcting this imbalance requires first an understanding of disease beyond its secular definition. When one understands the energies contained in both man and the universe, he is in a better position to understand disease and even to use disease itself to correct the problem. It may sound strange to say that one can "use" disease, but the best way to destroy an enemy is to understand its nature.

If everything in existence contains Divine life-will, how can that life-will be a part of imbalance or disease? Once again the Kabalist turns to the Tree of Life to understand this seeming distortion of God's will. Recall that man was created in the image and likeness of God. Therefore we must examine the Trees of Yetzirah and Assiah, the worlds of man/mankind, as they receive the impression/pattern for Divine life-will from the Worlds of Atziluth and Briah, God's worlds. Since Divine life and patterns are perfect and in balance, then it is obvious that they become distorted somewhere in the translation and transmission of that life and pattern through the worlds of man/mankind.

Figure 12.1 depicts the Worlds of Yetzirah and Assiah, as the former overlays the latter. Where the higher Tree overlays the lower, definitions of the centers that are above the line relate to the higher Tree of Yetzirah, and those below the line relate to the lower Tree of Assiah. These Trees relate to man and mankind, respectively. It bears repeating that, simply stated, Divine life-will or intent, meaning God or Divinity, is that origin or point from which the universe was emanated. It was the intent described in Genesis 1:2: "And the Spirit of God moved upon the face of the waters." That intent or life-will established the life-force that would empower the life of everything in existence, and established the life-form or pattern that everything would live in accordance with. "And God said [life-force], Let there be light [life-form] . . . ." We could say that these represent God's desire and God's intellect. In that brief statement all the life-force and life-form necessary to fulfill the life-will or intent for the creation was emanated. And although it is impossible to comprehend Divinity itself, remember that man was created in Divine image and likeness. Therefore it follows that those same principles are inherent in man. We could say that man was created to be a creator; it is his inherent nature.

An infant is born with the inherent capabilities of his parents. Those capabilities are demonstrated upon each level of

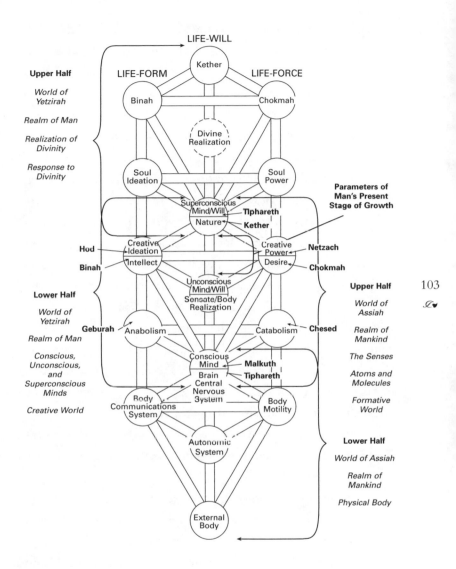

LIFE-WILL

Kether

LIFE-FORM

LIFE-FORCE

Binah

Chokmah

Divine
Realization

Soul
Ideation

Soul
Power

Superconscious
Mind/Will — **Tiphareth**

Nature — **Kether**

Creative
Ideation

Creative
Power — **Netzach**

Hod — Intellect

Desire — **Chokmah**

Binah

Unconscious
Mind/Will

Sensate/Body
Realization

Geburah — Anabolism

Catabolism — **Chesed**

Conscious
Mind — **Malkuth**

Brain
Central
Nervous
System — **Tiphareth**

Body
Communications
System

Body
Motility

Autonomic
System

External
Body

Upper Half

*World of
Yetzirah*

Realm of Man

*Realization of
Divinity*

*Response to
Divinity*

Lower Half

*World of
Yetzirah*

Realm of Man

*Conscious,
Unconscious,
and
Superconscious
Minds*

Creative World

**Parameters of
Man's Present
Stage of Growth**

Upper Half

*World of
Assiah*

*Realm of
Mankind*

The Senses

*Atoms and
Molecules*

*Formative
World*

Lower Half

World of Assiah

*Realm of
Mankind*

Physical Body

103

FIGURE 12.1. UNDERSTANDING DISEASE

growth from infancy through childhood and into adulthood. A child's parents may possess the blueprint of a house that the child will one day build. But until the child develops the ability to read the blueprint, use the tools, and construct the house, we could say that the ability to build a house is not fulfilled. Nonetheless, the growth process is absolutely necessary for the house to be built in accordance with its pattern. Errors are an important part of the growth process. They indicate the proper way of doing something, as well as allow the individual to integrate the understanding necessary for the proper application. Sometimes it is necessary to personify Divine life to better understand ourselves. Kabalah teaches that Divine life empowers everything in existence. Thus, when the awareness of the vessel that contains the consciousness increases, so does the empowerment of the inner Divine life. This is like saying the adults in our world are empowered by what their children accomplish, which we can certainly see in the results of technological and medical advancements. Each succeeding generation is also empowered in its growth process by such advancements. In like manner, man, through the growth experience, contributes to and further empowers Divinity, which is, of course, cycled back into the universe. This could be loosely termed "evolution."

In looking at figure 12.1, we see that life-will, life-force, and life-form descend into and through the world of man, who then transforms and transmits them into the world of mankind, his physical vehicle. Since the Divine pattern is undistorted and in balance, what happens in its transmission into the manifested world obviously occurs within man's transformation of that life. As has been stated previously, man has not kept pace with the evolutionary growth of the universe, so it could be said that he is attempting to build his house without having developed the ability to read the blueprint or use the tools. In the world of mankind, this results in physical and emotional ills or disease. Illness attempts to tell man that he needs to learn the proper procedure for building his house; when he does so, the distortions can be corrected and disease will not manifest in accordance with his personal pattern. However, we must also remember that there is not only personal but also collective distortion relative to mankind as a whole. Disease will not be eradicated in its entirety until everyone makes the necessary corrections. Everyone must build a proper house before the city will no longer evidence distortion.

Figure 12.1 illustrates the parameters within which man's current evolutionary growth is contained, and figuratively speaking, there is a very wide gap in ages as they relate to universal age. This is comparable to a college-level classroom in which the students' ages range from five to twenty, which would make for a none-too-successful study group. Any distortion that arose in such a study group would be demonstrated by the inability of the immature students to apply what they managed to learn from class. And so it is the same for disease in our world. Disease indicates man's inability to apply what he should have learned in the educational class of life; the awareness of this inability will allow us to utilize disease beneficially.

Reviewing the Tree, we see that there are two types of force flowing into existence. The first type is life-will, which descends from the Divine spark, called the monad, in Kether of Yetzirah, moves through Tiphareth of Yetzirah, and ends in either

105

Kether of Assiah, Nature, or Yesod of Yetzirah, the unconscious mind. This spark is the force that is transformed into inner strength, our capacity for experience during a life span. We can call this the will to exist, which is different from motivation. One can have the will to live, but little motivation to experience life. This will enlivens one's conscious will, as well as the unconscious will to exist. We can see this unconscious aspect of life-will at work in the body's autonomic system and in the "fight or flight" response of the animal nature within our essential self.

The second type of force is life-force, which descends from Chokmah of Yetzirah through Chesed of Yetzirah to Netzach of Yetzirah, its lowest frequency in the world of man, which is creative power, as it overlays and should govern Chokmah of Assiah, desire/motivation. Life-force energy must be contained in order to be viable; thus, the aspects of force upon the right pillar of the Tree are contained within and enliven the aspects of form upon the left pillar. The life-force of Netzach is contained within the form aspect of Hod, creative ideation, which overlays Binah of Assiah, intellect. Without containment, force dissipates. We see an example of life-force energy in its release from the food we eat, which then energizes the physical body.

Although life-will carries the intent for man's experience, if the aspects of life-force and life-form that life-will utilizes are imbalanced, then the final expression of that life-will will also be imbalanced. This imbalance will be evidenced within the physical and/or emotional levels of mankind. Thus life-force and life-form must be in balance with each other, and both must be expressed in accordance with balanced or proper life-will or intent.

Again looking at figure 12.1, you will note that the superconscious mind, or soul, Tiphareth of Yetzirah—the aspect of life-will that mankind should collectively express—overlays Kether of Assiah, the "God" of the World of Assiah, Nature. An example of the achievement of this status of will is the miracles described in the New Testament. This status of will in man is analogous on its level to that same level of will known as the physical body's will of metabolism. It is obvious that the Master Jesus had fully developed what we call the "metabolism" of His psyche, which impresses the "autonomic system" of the psyche to structure manifestation in accordance with the soul's intent. We hear the statement "we are one" many times, but just what does that mean? It means that in the adulthood of our expression, we—as the totality of man, the "man" created in God's image and likeness—are, from Divine perspective, one body. The recognition of this oneness becomes creative expression as man reaches his spiritual adulthood. This also causes us to realize that man, collectively, does indeed affect Nature. Earthquakes, tornadoes, storms, hurricanes, and so on all reflect the inner disturbances within the collective of mankind.

107

Superconscious will, Tiphareth of Yetzirah, uses the dual aspects of creative power—Netzach of Yetzirah—and creative ideation—Hod of Yetzirah—to establish what it intends. But because these aspects are identified with and governed by desire and intellect—Chokmah and Binah of Assiah, respectively— they respond to the unconscious will of Yesod of Yetzirah, as it is identified with and governed by sensate will, Daath of Assiah. The flow of will from Kether of Yetzirah never ceases, but when that flow is diverted into inappropriate channels that are not in accord with the highest intent or will of the superconscious mind within the human psyche, distortions are created by an unconscious mind that does not recognize the higher authority. The formative level then correctly follows the pattern given to it, but the pattern itself is incorrect.

The lowest aspect of will relating to man is conscious will, Malkuth of Yetzirah, which overlays and uses the brain, Tiphareth of Assiah. The brain can be wrong in its perception and the mind can be in error in its response to that perception. The conscious mind, through present experience, contributes to the reactive collective experience of the past in the unconscious mind. In this manner, the conscious mind can alter, enhance, or change the collective; however, it takes as much input energy to change an incorrect concept within the unconscious to a correct one as it did to instill the incorrect concept in the first place. Using higher healing frequencies, this change can be accomplished in a much shorter time. As the vibratory frequency of one's awareness increases, so too does empowerment, resulting in a more effective application of healing energy.

Just as the desire for that which is inappropriate for one's life experience can bring about unpleasant results, a distorted belief created by the intellect can also lead to the same. For an example of how creative ideation that is dominated by an incorrect intellectual concept can affect the body and produce a disturbance, consider a mother whose daughter is late coming home from school. Before she can ascertain why her child is late, the mother may begin to think that she has been in an accident, and the more she thinks about this, the more details she invents and incorporates into her new "truth." Soon the mother's body reacts to her new concept of truth: her heart beats faster, her nervous system begins to react, her stomach becomes upset, she feels the beginning of a headache, her blood pressure rises. Finally, as the body continues to react to this perception, the child arrives home and informs her mother that the teacher kept her after school to complete a certain task. With a sudden rush of relief, the force of anxiety is released from the form of what is now revealed as an "untruth," and the body returns to its normal state. This released force then often expresses itself in some form of reaction upon the physical level, as the mother expresses joy, love, and sometimes even anger at the child.

Now imagine a similar situation in which an incorrect concept has been held for long enough for the concept to become concrete and firmly set. The body vehicle would reflect that incorrect concept, since it is created in accordance with the patterns of which that concept is a part. An example of this type of distortion could be diabetes, a symptom of a misheld concept that life is bitter or unrewarding, which perhaps has continued for lifetimes. The correction of that concept becomes much more difficult, for unlike the arrival of the child, which relieved the symptoms, the individual must himself restructure the concept that has produced the distorted pattern.

In summary, the life-will of Spirit, or Divinity, is pure and in balance, but it becomes distorted as man receives its empowerment and then expresses it through a belief system and/or concepts that are no longer appropriate for his evolutionary age. That empowerment also shows itself through distorted or painful life experiences that are designed to indicate the next "lesson" in life, or to indicate a latent principle that the individual is now capable of developing. When we understand disease

109

and take action to either correct the concept or develop the principle, then the distortion can be corrected.

Another important aspect regarding disease is to understand the need for the release of consciousness from the physical body—death—when the body is beyond the capability of being healed. Man must change his attitude regarding death, for often man's fear of death leads to his taking desperate measures in fighting disease, when it would be better to try to understand why disease is occurring. Man must learn to dissociate himself from his identification with his body. He must not only intellectually comprehend but integrate the understanding that life goes on in one form or another, and that the quality of life is more important than the quantity. Death is the release of consciousness from a body that is no longer viable, giving consciousness a chance to renew itself into a new form not as incapacitated as the old one. Death is a renewal, not a loss, but until man accepts this as part of his reality, he will continue to experience pain and loss far beyond its necessity.

Although scientific research is important, and one would be very foolish not to take full advantage of every form of healing available, man must reach a point where he also takes full responsibility for his own health. He must reverse his viewpoint that disease is an enemy to be met, fought, and conquered and begin to treat disease as the friend that it is. Disease, in a sense, is actually the life-will of God forming the resistance or "light" by which we can realize that aspect within ourselves. As previously stated, just as pain is a symptom of disease, disease is a symptom of an inner disharmony creating a distorted pattern, which, in turn, allows the disease to manifest.

13

Causes of Disease

As stated previously, disease exists within all kingdoms and is governed by the law of cause and effect in its cycling of vertical energies within the totality of man/mankind. It always promotes liberation and is designed to either correct a concept of creative expression or integrate a certain attribute. In short, disease represents a lack of harmony within man, the inner being; when disease is grounded into the outer being, mankind, it is made evident in emotional or physical disharmony.

To review, there are three major areas related to disease that also relate to those pillars of the Tree of Life representing life-will, life-force, and life-form. The area of life-will affects the heart, circulatory system, and nervous system; the area of life-force affects respiration; and the area of life-form affects assimilation and elimination. Certain diseases can be termed "regional"; that is, they affect many, and sometimes all, parts of the body. These diseases usually represent an accumulation of lesser distortions from prior evolutionary life—in other words, from many lifetimes. The lesser symptoms or indications of distortion finally lead to a far greater and widespread distortion. Examples of regional diseases are cancer, tumors, arthritis, and skin problems. Some regional diseases, although centered in a specific part of the body, still greatly affect the body's overall efficiency.

There are five kinds of disease:

1. disease arising out of a physical, emotional/ intellectual, or creative condition that is inherited from one's evolutionary past;
2. disease to which all people are prone but need a predisposition in order to manifest;
3. disease in which one succumbs to infection or contagion;
4. disease inherent in the soil;
5. disease that occurs from overemphasis on a certain aspect of one's life.

To understand the first kind of disease, let us use an analogy. A child begins to attend school, and for whatever reason chooses not to learn to read. If he is promoted to higher grades, his inability to read becomes more problematic, and the distortion caused by this inability becomes more prominent. Should the child either leave school or graduate without having learned to read, his entire life experience would become distorted, or, we could say, diseased. Remember that, as children of God, we are also growing from infancy to adulthood within our evolutionary life span, our goal being to continuously develop those innate principles of expression that compose the reality of our being. As we advance to each successive stage of growth, the distortions that were not very noticeable in the earlier stages become much more evident in the later stages. Contrary to appearances, this is not a punishment but a blessing. By examining our emotional/physical distortions, we can discover which principle needs to be developed and/or strengthened. Following the aphorism "as above, so below" or "as within, so without," we recognize that we are indeed children of God, but just as our offspring grow up, we cannot remain spiritual children. The universal mandate of God's nature is continued growth, which requires the integration of those "subjects" (principles) that are essential for spiritual maturity.

The concepts that were learned during man's childhood are often inappropriate for his adulthood. But because man has not integrated the concepts (lessons) necessary for his adult expression, he, like the child who never learned to read, faces tremendous insecurity and fear of assuming the responsibility of his adult life. Thus fear and insecurity empower inappropriate childhood concepts with the strength of an adult consciousness, resulting in the many diseases that run rampant in our world. Consequently, it is important to discover the concepts that are producing the emotional/physical distortion or disease. This may require therapeutic counseling with a professional who is trained to reveal emotional experiences and beliefs that negatively affect an individual's life experience.

Therapeutic investigation often looks to the past, the childhood, to identify those concepts that did not originate there but were a part of an individual's inherent makeup before he was born into his family. Mysticism teaches that childhood experiences do

113

not make us what we are, but that we are "magnetically" drawn to the families and experiences that are appropriate for our next stage of growth. A therapist can aid an individual by defining the predominant concepts evidenced in childhood that later affect one's adult life. However, unless the improper concepts are replaced by appropriate ones, they will simply return. Integration of correct concepts goes far beyond simple intellectual definition, although definition is the first and important step in the process. Kabalistic healing can be a powerful adjunct to this process, as will be seen later in this book.

Let us now investigate the predisposition to a disease, or what is often called a genetic predisposition. The genes that compose an individual's makeup reflect whether the individual is prone to a particular disease. First, the question must be asked, what creates the genes? Being physically tangible, genes are the final result of a higher pattern, a pattern carried forward into each life by the unconscious mind. This pattern was drawn into physical existence through a body, which would reflect that pattern genetically. In other words, the predisposition did not come to the individual; the individual came to the predisposition by virtue of the pattern for his life experience.

Returning to the example of learning to read, consider a child who comes from a family in which no one has learned to read. The longer the child holds fast to the belief that he, too, can never learn to read, the more he reinforces his inability. But if he faces the task of learning to read with confidence and applies himself to it, he will never encounter the distortion and pain of illiteracy. The child has a choice of which path to take when faced with the task of learning to read. If he chooses to reinforce the inability, as his family has, he strengthens his incorrect belief or concept.

Now let us use predisposition to cancer as an example. Cancer usually manifests where there has been an established pattern of intolerance, crystallization, and/or prejudice, or where there is a need to integrate tolerance, flexibility, self-nurturing, and acceptance. These latter qualities are not necessarily manifested in a negative sense, but may now be appropriate for integration by the individual. For the cancer to be eliminated, either the negative quality must be transmuted or the positive quality integrated. In the case of breast cancer, for instance, these qualities might be related to nurturing, either lacking in oneself or improperly expressed to another. If the individual does not begin to correct the pattern, the predisposition for cancer will probably manifest in the disease.

115

How this manifestation happens is an example of how intellect, vitalized by life-force, can produce a pattern from the seed already planted within the genes of the individual. A woman may say, "My grandmother had breast cancer, my mother had breast cancer, and so I will probably have breast cancer." As she grows older, the fear becomes greater and, in a sense, acts as fertilizer enabling that seed of belief to actually grow and produce exactly what she expected. Remember that fear is a binding force that draws to itself that which is feared; through fear, one can actually create disease. But if this woman were to examine her experience and try to integrate what the disease she feared was endeavoring to tell her, the disease could be avoided. If she were to look back on family history and discover the similarity of expressions in her grandmother and in her mother, she would see the qualities referenced by the disease in herself, and she could correct the pattern.

Cancer itself represents unabridged and uncontrolled cells. "As above, so below," and vice versa; if the cells are out of control, then so is the pattern held within the mind for their expression in whatever area the problem exists. Cells out of control in breast cancer indicate intolerance or prejudice in relationship to what one nurtures. An example of this is a mother who is so prejudiced toward her child that she would go to any length to further what she believes to be the child's best interests, even to the point of manipulating the child into adopting the same beliefs. Another case would be a woman who never nurtures herself, and is intolerant of her own interests to the point of neglecting her own growth while constantly serving others. There is nothing wrong with service to others, but it should never result from the denial of one's own spirit or be motivated by the need to reinforce one's self-importance.

Succumbing to infection or contagion, the third type of disease, results from the inability to destroy the microbes causing them or from an immune deficiency. As discussed earlier, immunity is directly related to the heart center, Tiphareth, upon the Tree of Life. This center is the Self referred to by Jung; and being the heart or core of one's existence, it relates directly to self-identity, self-worth, and self-love, particularly as these qualities become the intent for the dual force and form of Netzach and Hod of the Tree, whose virtues are selflessness and truthfulness, respectively. These virtues apply to oneself just as easily as one applies them to the life experience. To ensure the strength achieved by self-identity, one must be honest with oneself and endeavor to live his life for the betterment of all humanity, rather than out of a grasping, fearful selfishness without regard for anyone else. The degree to which one has established the certainty of his being is the degree of his immunity to disease. Such certainty is not based on external accomplishments, possessions, or titles, which are defined by the vice of Tiphareth, pride. The certainty of being could be demonstrated as faith, joy, or confidence, but even these all fall short of truly explaining a state of existence in which one establishes peace and balance within the life experience.

The heart center relates to the thymus, and the use of its energy can promote additional immunity. An example of this is those instances where doctors and nurses worked unselfishly with those afflicted with the plague, yet never developed the disease. With the recognition and acceptance of one's true identity, the heart center is stimulated; but the opposite of this, a lack of even external self-worth, is prevalent in our world today, with its logical outcome of a decrease in immunity.

An individual suffering a disease caused by immune deficiency can greatly stimulate his own immunity by devoting energy to the betterment of others. The virtue of Tiphareth, devotion to the Great Work, means living one's life for the purpose of the enhancement of all life. The result of such devotion is that one does not feed the disease or add to its intensity. One should acknowledge the disease, provide containment for it, and seek whatever medical help he deems appropriate, but then should direct his life-force energy elsewhere, depriving the disease of that energy. What usually occurs is that an individual directs all of his life-force and conscious existence in an endeavor to simply stay alive. However, in doing so he creates the disease as his identity—so that his life becomes the disease.

An individual who has a disease must accept the fact that from the highest level of his being, he has created his present circumstances, and that he can wallow in them or rise above them—the choice is his. The greatest help comes only from within him, and Kabalistic healing techniques can help empower and strengthen the individual's inner development, as well as address the physical aspect of the condition. Through these applications, some form of healing will occur, but one must not expect instant results to be seen within the body itself. "Instant cures" and "miracles" are sometimes seen if the intended level of understanding is attained, dependent upon each individual's own pattern for life. However, the purpose of all healing on any level is to help the individual achieve a state of harmony in which pattern distortions may be corrected by that individual's own awareness.

Mankind must also acquire an understanding of the aspect we call "death," for it is often the fear of death that causes even more emphasis to be placed on curing disease; so much so, in fact, that the disease becomes the individual's identity. It is also important to understand that a full cure for a disease is possible, but may not be probable. What is accomplished in the quality of life prior to death is part of a continuing evolutionary life span; thus the quality of life attained becomes the foundation upon which the next life is built.

Some systems of thought that deal with healing disease claim that if you do A, B, and C, you will be cured. The individual who does A, B, and C and is not cured often believes that he has in some way failed, which only adds to the insecurity. A, B, and C may add to the correction of the distorted pattern, but if the distortion requires more energy for correction than is capable of being exerted in the remainder of this lifetime—or if the body vehicle is beyond repair—a full cure cannot be effected, even though great strides can be made. What is of most importance is what can be accomplished in the time allotted. One should certainly express the desire to be healed, but not be so deeply immersed within that desire that an unfulfilled expectation will create even more distortion.

The fourth cause of disease is inherent in the soil. This refers to the microbes contained in the physical vehicle of mankind that, upon burial, are returned to the earth itself; it also refers to the consciousness that has existed within every cell of that body and which belongs to the totality of consciousness of collective humanity. It has been stated that the viruses that attack mankind are, in reality, the antibodies created by collective humanity to destroy the imbalance or disease man inflicts on the earth. This is akin to fighting fire with fire. Viruses are created by an intelligence, but whose intelligence could this be, other than that of collective humanity? Cancer cells can be said to be distorted, and yet as cells they are perfect; they simply follow the pattern set for them. Only the pattern is distorted. Some feel that mankind has become a cancer upon the earth, an argument that makes sense when one compares the four World Trees of man to the beauty and balance of the Universal Tree of Life. We are cells running rampant, perfectly following a distorted pattern and creating chaos on the earth over which man was given dominion. The body of the earth gives back to mankind the manifestation of those distorted patterns in the form of microbes and bacteria that are not conducive to mankind's life; but it was man's creativity that established the patterns upon which they are based.

The fifth cause of disease results from overemphasizing a certain principle or aspect in one's life to the point that it produces an imbalance within the psyche of man, resulting in either emotional or physical disease. This can happen even in the life of one who is so devoted to a spiritual growth process that a balanced life appropriate for such growth cannot be expressed. We could use the term *fanatic* to describe such a person. An overemphasis on any principle will result in its opposite polarity. For instance, an overemphasis on love can produce "smother love" and a myriad of negative feelings. In many cases one loses his individualism and becomes that which he is so focused on, completely identifying with it.

The causes of disease given in this chapter are a generalization, much as there is a generalization of the understanding of medicine. Like physicians, however, those who work in the healing field must establish a far wider understanding of these causes in order to help others reach an understanding that applies to their individual levels. This understanding is not reached by merely reading a book, any more than reading *Gray's Anatomy* entitles one to practice medicine. It can, however, be acquired by effort, dedication, and practice by one with a desire to serve mankind.

14

The Evolution
of Disease

Just as man's consciousness has evolved, as evidenced by our current level of technological sophistication, we must realize that the consciousness of disease grows and evolves at the same time. It changes its form of manifestation in accordance with man's level of awareness. Man's mental/creative processes are responsible for what seems to be the eradication of certain diseases. But while man has been successful in eradicating the form of diseases, he cannot destroy the consciousness that occupied these forms. Like man's consciousness, disease consciousness can only be transmuted; thus the consciousness of diseases will continue to evolve and, like man, utilize ever more refined forms.

We must remember that the energy of a disease, its consciousness, is force assuming some kind of form. When that force is blocked or halted in one type of form, it will manifest within a newer form, until man learns the lesson that disease is endeavoring to indicate.

Esoteric philosophy has long described five major diseases that continue to affect mankind: tuberculosis, social diseases (such as syphilis and gonorrhea), cancer, heart diseases, and nervous system diseases. Powerful drugs have been discovered that appear to have conquered many of these diseases, particularly tuberculosis, syphilis, and gonorrhea. These drugs give the appearance of having won the battle, but the war wages on, because the consciousnesses of these diseases evolve into more highly resistant strains or become incorporated into other diseases that allow them to exist. Meanwhile, the pattern for such diseases as cancer, heart disease, and nervous system disease establishes itself even more strongly within the collective consciousness of mankind, as these diseases become much more prevalent.

Tuberculosis, for instance, was believed to be eradicated, but we now see it surfacing in strains that no longer respond to previous drug treatment, and we also see it finding a freedom of expression in AIDS. In fact, AIDS has become a field of activity for most of the major diseases we've listed. One wonders, Where does it stop? Man is faced with "fighting" what allows the manifestation of other diseases, rather than the diseases themselves. The forms of pneumocystic pneumonia (like tuberculosis, affecting the lungs) and Kaposi's sarcoma cancer (cells running rampant) are very rare diseases that man, at present, has great difficulty in overcoming. Also, AIDS can be acquired from two of the most prevalent expressions of negative energy in society today: drug use and promiscuous sex.

If man had heeded what the existence of syphilis and gonorrhea indicated—as they represented a distortion in man's expression of his innate principles—we might not be dealing today with AIDS, which, by destroying the T-helper cells, affects man's ability to produce immunity to many diseases and infections. Cancer is on the upswing, and while blame may be placed in some part upon the environment, we must look beyond environment to another source: the collective consciousness of mankind. Mankind, like cancerous cells running rampant, is continually augmenting the vices of those principles of Netzach and Hod that relate directly to his created existence. These vices are lust, misused life-force, promiscuity, falsehood, dishonesty, and criticism, all of which seem to dominate the world of man's existence.

123

In one sense, the higher Self within man, Tiphareth of Yetzirah, is impressing its powerful will or intent for development upon Nature, Kether of Assiah, in that lower World, producing the distortions or disease whose inappropriateness for a harmonious life indicates the lessons (principles) that are necessary for that development. By destroying the form, man allows it to evolve into stronger and more refined bodies. The only way to cease this vicious cycle is to begin to develop those attributes or principles that the disease indicates are lacking. Man must begin to investigate the reason for disease occurring in its present form, along with doing what is necessary to alleviate the disease itself.

To do this requires use of the intellect, as well as a desire for personal inner growth. Along with mental/creative efforts expended to discover a cure for a disease, man must begin to examine his own intellectual/emotional level and remember that not only those affected by a disease must do this, but all mankind as well, since we are all affected by the collective consciousness. Each person is responsible not only for his portion but also for the totality.

Nature—Kether of Assiah, the God of that World—is issued a mandate through man's own potential to express a form of disease by which man is to integrate the understanding of God's laws, thereby developing the principles of his own inner being. It is rather sad, then, that man deceives himself by thinking that in the long run he can prevent disharmony through use of his own imbalanced and undeveloped divine nature, or that he thinks he can ever hope to outwit God as Nature. It would be of great benefit, and certainly much less painful, if man would begin to reach within for the reasons behind disease and pain.

We must give credit to science and medicine for the strides made in alleviating disease; however, unless man begins to investigate the deeper understanding of the occurrence of disease, it is much like putting out small fires while ignoring the source of the flames. The intent to relieve man's pain is commendable, but in actuality only man can eradicate the consciousness that takes the form of disease—not by eliminating that consciousness, but by transmuting it into the understanding it has been created to present.

The resistance of some diseases to certain antibiotics is simply the evolutionary strength their consciousnesses have developed through the successive forms they have taken. Remember that the disease itself is in accordance with its correct pattern, a pattern formulated by man in accordance with his status and needs. Anything that threatens the existence of disease is its enemy, an enemy it will constantly endeavor to defeat. Only man, the creator of the pattern for the disease, can change it. In a sense, destroying the form disease takes strengthens it, endowing it with a newer and better vehicle for its expression.

We certainly must utilize what science and medicine have developed, but we must also make the inner effort to understand disease if we wish to see it completely eradicated. Mankind's suffering is due partly to his misunderstanding of the law of nonresistance, his attitude and fear regarding death, and his feeling that disappearance of the form of his body indicates disaster.

The law of nonresistance is the acceptance of things as they are, while endeavoring to correct disturbances and distortions from the pattern within upon which they are based. One must restructure his outer world from within, for it is the "within" that has created it.

15

The Totality of Man/Mankind upon the Trees of Yetzirah and Assiah

Having been created in God's (World of Atziluth) image (World of Briah), man (World of Yetzirah) then creates mankind (World of Assiah) in man's image. That image then arises out of man's thought and is impressed upon man's creative ability, which establishes a form complying with the pattern of that thought. Man and man's vehicle, mankind, are interdependent; that is to say, each depends upon the other for life experience. When the evolutionary cycle of life began, it was necessary for man, the mind-being, to achieve the understanding of his body, or vehicle, and the external world, so that he would gradually achieve dominion over them relative to each level of growth. This is like a child who, by virtue of his growth and experiences, develops greater strength and responsibility relative to each stage of growth. The purpose of the child's first stage of growth, however, is to become acquainted and familiar with his world. The toys and games of childhood are "practice" for his future adult status.

The consciousness of man as a mind-being has, in its evolutionary growth, ascended through the world of mankind, enabling it to become acquainted and familiar with that world. Consequently, when man reaches spiritual adulthood, his consciousness should be able to govern that world in an appropriate manner. (The story of this transition from childhood to adulthood is described in the Genesis narrative of Jacob and Esau.) However, man has already developed the strength associated with adulthood but has retained the beliefs and concepts of his childhood. The outcome is a distorted world, one that is out of balance in many areas but the distortion of which is especially evident in disease.

To understand man, we must also understand mankind, since the relationship between them comprises two aspects of one totality in life. Mankind cannot function without the intent of the mind to direct it, and man could not exist without that which responds to the directives of the mind within the life experience. Figure 15.1 places the entirety of man/mankind upon those Worlds of Yetzirah and Assiah, formerly labeled man's and mankind's worlds. Nothing in the universe is separate or distinct from everything else. The overlaying of Yetzirah and Assiah indicates the interaction between man and mankind and their worlds—active, formative, creative, and spiritual. You will note that man's creative world overlays mankind's formative world, which indicates that man's creative ability directs mankind's formative

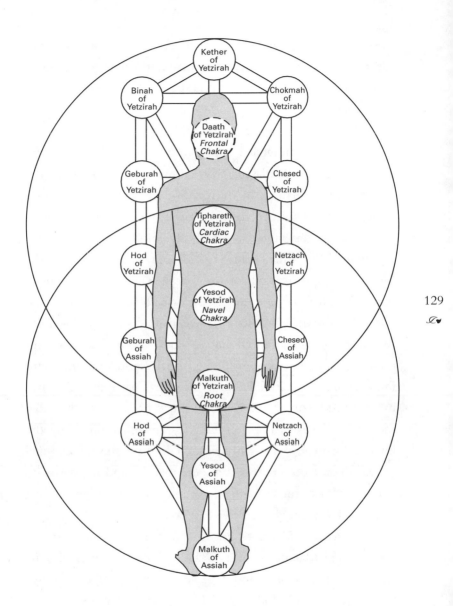

129

FIGURE 15.1. THE TOTALITY OR ENTIRETY OF
MAN/MANKIND ON THE TREES OF YETZIRAH/ASSIAH

world of the senses, atoms, and molecules into action and form. Although we separated man and mankind for the purpose of understanding each of them, we must consider them as a totality in experience.

Just as man interacts with mankind through the overlaying of the Trees of Yetzirah and Assiah, Divinity interacts with man through the overlaying of the lower half of Briah on the upper half of Yetzirah. In the division of man/mankind into three sectors—active, formative/creative, and spiritual—we have found the esoteric reference to body, mind, and Spirit commonly used. Since the creative world of the mind(s) overlays the formative world of mankind, we can then say that the mind is the creator. It formulates the image or pattern that is impressed upon the formative "substance," which results in manifestation. In much the same way, Divinity's "conscious and unconscious minds" are impressed upon the spiritual world of man. If this impression were faithfully reproduced by man's thought, harmony would exist in the world. Again it becomes evident that the problem lies in the domination of man's thought by the intellect, desire, and senses of mankind. In short, this is the refusal of man's consciousness to assume the identity and responsibility that accord with the strength of its adult status. We might say that man exhibits a "universal Peter Pan complex."

In figure 15.1, note that the feet of man/mankind are placed upon Malkuth of Assiah, the Sephirah of external existence, which man/mankind experiences through life. Next we have Netzach and Hod of Assiah supporting that existence as they relate to Yesod of that World, the inner strength of the body as it is kept in balance and maintained through the autonomic, motility, and communication systems. The first overlaying of the Trees' Sephiroth occurs at Tiphareth of Assiah, the brain and central nervous system of mankind, which is overlaid by Malkuth of Yetzirah, man's conscious mind. Herein is transmitted the intent for life experience. Responding to the intent, though not directly impacted by any Sephiroth from the higher World, Chesed and Geburah of Assiah—the metabolic aspects of catabolism and anabolism—govern the storage and release of body energy. A great deal can be understood in studying man's evolution according to this interaction of Trees; however, we are using only a brief simplification as it applies to Kabalistic healing. Malkuth of Yetzirah is also the Sephirah on the Tree associated with the root chakra, which, along with the other chakras, will be discussed in the following chapter. This chakra represents man's grounding within the past experience of mankind and the procreative instinct that enabled the continuation of mankind.

The next higher level of connection in figure 15.1 is between Yesod of Yetzirah, the unconscious mind, and Daath of Assiah, which Yesod overlays. Daath of Assiah is the body's realization of itself in its response to the senses that govern it. In addition, as they relate to the body's functions, the senses also interact with the body's metabolism, ensuring that the body continues to function properly. As discussed previously, the unconscious mind, Yesod of Yetzirah, is the repository for the reactions relative to all past experience of man and represents the navel chakra, also known as the solar plexus. Being the intent of will for creative functioning, Yesod of Yetzirah should be governed by Hod (creative ideation) and Netzach (creative power), but as long as it is identified with the sensate realization of Daath of Assiah, it is dominated by Binah and Chokmah of Assiah—intellect and desire, respectively. Being overlaid by Hod and Netzach of Yetzirah, Binah and Chokmah should be directed by them rather than dominating them. The ruling authority of the creative/formative world is Yesod of Yetzirah as it overlays Daath of Assiah. By way of metaphor, we could say that Daath of Assiah is the epitome of childhood growth, while Yesod of Yetzirah is the teenage stage of transition from childhood to adulthood, an adulthood that is represented by the next higher Sephirah of the Tree, Tiphareth of Yetzirah.

Tiphareth of Yetzirah is the superconscious mind, also called the soul, and it overlays the "God" of Assiah, Kether. Interestingly, the superconscious mind is itself overlaid by Malkuth of Briah, or, one might say, the "conscious mind" of Divinity. Thus only through the superconscious or soul can direct contact be made with the next higher level of Divine intent. Superconscious mind represents the adult spiritual expressive nature for the sensate/physical world. Tiphareth of Yetzirah directs those principles of Hod and Netzach of its World; however, if those principles are dominated by the sensate world's desire and intellect, Binah and Chokmah of Assiah, they become unsuitable for the expression relative to the adult status of spirituality. This would be akin to a physician attempting to use a child's "doctor kit" to treat his patients.

Tiphareth represents the heart, or cardiac chakra, and like the heart within mankind, the cardiac chakra becomes the core or center of the totality of man/mankind. Tiphareth of Yetzirah draws upon Chesed and Geburah of that World for the patterns relative to its intent. Next, those patterns are transmitted down to Netzach and Hod of Yetzirah, which are most often unable to interpret them into the childlike world of the unconscious mind. This would be like giving a three-year-old a medical kit and asking that child to treat patients with real illnesses. Chesed and Geburah represent what has been accrued relative to spiritual adult status, but if nothing has been accrued then there is nothing for Tiphareth to draw upon to fulfill its intent. Its will is then impressed upon inappropriate childlike principles, which in turn create disease and/or distortion in the physical body in order to indicate what is lacking in the developmental process. Like Chesed and Geburah of Assiah, Chesed and Geburah of Yetzirah are autonomous in their World.

The highest chakra of man that is represented by a middle pillar Sephirah on the Tree is Daath of Yetzirah, which does not overlay any Sephirah in the lower World but is overlaid by Yesod of Briah—what one could call the "unconscious mind" of Divinity. Daath of Yetzirah eventually becomes to man what Daath of Assiah is to mankind: the realization of himself as a mind-being who, through that realization, establishes himself as a cocreator with Divinity. That, however, will occur during the next stage of growth, after man has identified himself as the mind-being he is and completed the evolutionary educational process appropriate for that status. Daath of Yetzirah represents the brow, or frontal chakra, often called the "third eye." It is a singular eye, since it does not need duality to determine its proper expression; it simply knows what is in accord with Divine will and expression.

Encircled in the diagram are those worlds of man and mankind, Yetzirah and Assiah, as well as a third aspect wherein the worlds of man and mankind interact. We could say that this stage indicates the transitional time from the childhood of mankind to the adulthood of man, a time similar to the teenage stage of life. What was developed during the teen years is not lost when one becomes an adult, but rather is empowered and refined due to the development of a higher awareness. The heart, or core, of this aspect of man/mankind is Yesod of Yetzirah as it overlays Daath of Assiah, the will of the unconscious mind as it expresses through sensate realization. What has been gained from the growth process of childhood (Yesod) must begin to respond to adult concepts and responsibility (Tiphareth). This cannot occur if the sensate realization of childhood continues to dominate what has been acquired from the educational process of growth.

134

The teenage stage is the shortest stage of growth, and yet it is often the most intense and active, a difficult time of transition from childhood to adulthood. The teenager lives in two worlds, just as a consciousness centered within the unconscious mind lives in both the world of mankind and the world of man. If the teenager continues to identify himself as a child, his gradual growth into adulthood will be governed by his childhood impressions, including the educational process so vital to adult expression.

At one time, man was meant to experience the "teen" years of his evolutionary growth. But now, however, he should be living his years of spiritual adulthood while expressing the results of his educational process with the strength of that adulthood. Instead, he is still creating his life based on the childhood images and fantasies he should have discarded during those teen years. From the survival instinct of Malkuth to the gut-feeling nature of Yesod, man should now be developing the intuitional (knowing) nature of the Self—Tiphareth—and, as a result, complying with Tiphareth's virtue of devotion to the Great Work, as each pattern within that Great Work is impressed upon the heart of man by Divine consciousness.

16

The Chakras

Figure 15.1 depicted the Sephiroth of the middle pillar of the Yetziratic Tree of man as they symbolized four of the energy centers, or chakras, within man. Since there are essentially seven chakras to which we currently relate, the additional three chakras would be placed on the three pathways that connect the side pillar Sephiroth. Figure 16.1 depicts all seven major energy centers essential for man's interaction with his vehicle for expression, mankind.

The word *chakra* is derived from Sanskrit and means "wheel" or "whirling disc." These energy centers have been known in esoteric understanding dating as far back as the Vedic texts. Many clairvoyants have attempted to describe how they appear, but each pictorial definition is in accord only with the viewpoint and perspective of the describer. What those descriptions represent is of

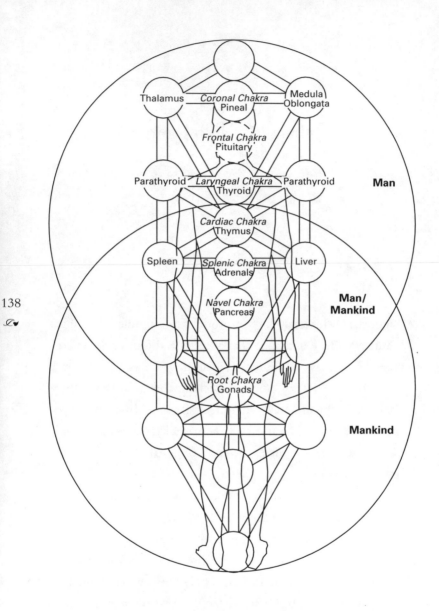

Man

Man/
Mankind

Mankind

Thalamus · *Coronal Chakra* Pineal · Medula Oblongata

Frontal Chakra Pituitary

Parathyroid · *Laryngeal Chakra* Thyroid · Parathyroid

Cardiac Chakra Thymus

Spleen · *Splenic Chakra* Adrenals · Liver

Navel Chakra Pancreas

Root Chakra Gonads

FIGURE 16.1. THE CHAKRAS ON THE TREES
OF MAN/MANKIND'S WORLDS

far greater importance than how they actually look, because intangible energies always take their form in accordance with the "eye" of the beholder.

When placed upon the Trees of man/mankind's worlds, Yetzirah and Assiah, the chakras extend no lower than Malkuth of Yetzirah overlaying Tiphareth of Assiah. The lower half of the World of Assiah belongs to mankind's physical body as it is governed and directed by the brain and central nervous system. The highest chakra within the world of man is placed at the juncture of a horizontal path between Chokmah and Binah and a vertical path between Kether and Daath. This is known as the coronal, or crown, chakra into which is received the impulse of Kether of Yetzirah, man's own innate spirit. This chakra is termed the "Crown."

Two other chakras are also formed at the juncture of horizontal and vertical paths. The laryngeal, or throat, chakra is at the juncture of the path joining Chesed and Geburah of Yetzirah and the path where Daath and Tiphareth meet. The splenic, or spleen, chakra is at the juncture of the path joining Netzach and Hod of Yetzirah and the path joining Tiphareth and Yesod. Where horizontal paths and vertical paths meet, powerful vortices of energy are created that interact with those centers of will established upon the middle pillar of the Tree.

The work of the chakras is twofold. First, they absorb and distribute prana, or vitality, to the physical body through the body's magnetic field, called the etheric double. Second, the chakras direct into mankind's consciousness those principles and their qualities that are developed within man. We could say that they transmit the level of man's growth into mankind's existence.

This second aspect is often related to the development of the force known as "kundalini," which is simply the grounding of man's innate Divine spirit into evolutionary life, together with its subsequent continued growth and empowerment. Each stage of a human life brings forth the capability of exhibiting certain qualities, the will relating to that stage being the empowerment of intent for the same. The will of kundalini that rises in mankind enables that vehicle to respond to the evolving will of man. Because kundalini is the essence of the pure force of God as it is grounded into manifestation within man/mankind, as well as the pure force of God that created the universe, it is that same pure force instilled within man that enables him to develop himself as a cocreator with God within his own personal/collective universe.

To apply these concepts to Kabalistic healing, we will first discuss the chakras as they transmit prana to the physical realm. Prana is one of the three forces necessary for man's existence. The other two are fohat—the primal force of will that emanates into all interchangeable physical forces, such as electricity, motion, heat, sound, and magnetism—and kundalini, the feminine force of Divinity contained within man/mankind. Among the Divine Trinity of the Tree, fohat aligns with Kether, prana with Chokmah, and kundalini with Binah.

Prana is considered the energy of the sun conveyed to the physical body through the breathing process, as well as by the chakras as they absorb and distribute this life-force to the intangible level of the senses, atoms, and molecules, and from there to the tangible level of the body. The chakras are vortices of energy often described as saucerlike depressions of varying sizes and brightness corresponding to the development of the individual.

The energy transmitted by the chakras enters into mankind's physical body through one of the endocrine or ductless glands to which it is attached by a stem of energy. Prana enters into the center of each chakra from the higher level and then radiates out from that center, much like the spokes of a wheel. The movement of the downward force into the chakra sets up a secondary movement of force that spins around the chakra while passing over and under the spokes in a weaving motion.

The chakras are located along the spinal column, and the stems that connect the chakras to the endocrine glands pass through the spine. It is through the endocrine glands that messages to the various parts of the body are conveyed. The endocrine glands secrete into the blood certain hormones that act as messengers, regulating and integrating body functions. The endocrine or ductless glands work closely with the three major duct glands of the body: the heart, liver, and spleen.

Figure 16.1 depicts the chakras and glands in relationship to man's interaction with mankind as symbolized by the Tree of Life. The principles of the Sephiroth are expressed—relative to man's spiritual age—through the vehicle of mankind, impacting the glands responsible for receiving the patterns of that expression into the intangible realm of mankind. In turn, this brings about either balance or distortion within the physical body. An analogy can be seen in the case of a man who is hard of hearing: Because of his inability to hear correctly, his attempt to repeat what someone else said might result in a distortion. That distortion would reflect the inability of the listener to hear clearly. When distortions are evident in the physical body, it is often because the level from which the body is maintained cannot "hear" correctly. The distortion can indicate not only the problem but also the probable cause. Remember that this impact applies to activity expressed from man to mankind that reflects that expression. An imbalance in the activity reflects itself into the activity of those glands and organs relative to the level of expression.

The first chakra in the ascent of the chakras upon the Tree is the root, or basic, chakra, lying at the base of the spine. It transmits patterned life-force energy to the gonads within the male and female reproductive systems. This chakra, through energizing the sexual nature, is necessary for procreation. It is also believed to aid in the maintenance of heat within the physical body. The root chakra is represented by Malkuth upon the Yetziratic Tree.

The second chakra is known as the navel, or umbilical, chakra, and the gland receiving its influence is the pancreas. This chakra is represented by Yetziratic Yesod, the foundation for existence. It is also known as the solar plexus, the source of power for the autonomic system of the body. The navel chakra is associated with feelings and emotions and is the connection to mankind's basic animal nature. When an individual says he has a "gut feeling" and refers to the area of the solar plexus, it is an indication that the feeling arises out of his animal, instinctual nature. This feeling may serve a purpose, but it is important to understand that it is not derived from a very high level of awareness. It is now time for man to rise from "feeling" to "knowing." The pancreas, to which the energy from the navel chakra flows, regulates sugar content in the blood, which, in turn, flows through the liver, providing body heat and energy. Esoterically, the pancreas relates to power, power representing basic strength.

The third chakra, known as the spleen, or splenic, chakra, lies on the horizontal path joining Netzach (creative power) and Hod (ideation) where it is intersected by the vertical path between Tiphareth and Yesod that joins the Sephiroth representing the navel and cardiac chakras. The splenic chakra works closely with the liver and spleen, while it focuses its energy through the adrenals. The splenic chakra absorbs vitality from the atmosphere, disintegrates the energy, and then transmutes prana to the various parts of the body. Prana gives life to the dense and subtle levels of mankind and affects the degree of health of those parts in accordance with the amount of prana distributed. Also important is the fact that the adrenals are the fighters within the endocrine chain. They maintain salt and water content within the blood and are essential to the synthesis of glycogen by the voluntary muscles. The adrenals secrete a hormone that raises blood pressure and increases the heart rate, thereby acting as a vascular and cardiac stimulant. They also affect the autonomic system and the heart through their hormones.

143

The liver, a component aspect of the splenic chakra, helps generate blood, eliminates toxins, secretes bile, stores carbohydrates, and changes proteins. The liver, represented by Yetziratic Netzach, is considered the gateway to the desire nature that is evidenced by the fact that Netzach of Yetzirah overlays Chokmah of Assiah, mankind's principle of desire/motivation. Thus, the liver carries tremendous emotional force, and the emotional status of the body affects it greatly. The spleen, the other dual component of the splenic chakra, is represented by Hod of Yetzirah. It holds within it susceptibility and resistance to the destruction of form. It is responsible for the manufacture and renewal of the cellular elements within the blood, and it eliminates worn-out materials. The substance known as ectoplasm is manufactured through the spleen. Ectoplasm was that which mediums used to formulate a vehicle for discarnate entities.

The fourth chakra is the heart, or cardiac, chakra, represented by Tiphareth of Yetzirah. The heart is the central core of the body, and the heart chakra is the core or hub between the worlds of Divinity and the worlds of man and mankind. The heart is the motor that continuously pumps the life-essence of the blood throughout the body. In the heart, the life-will principle of man blends with the blood. The blood also carries hormones, messengers from the ductless glands, that regulate and integrate body functions. It is blood, then, that regulates the nervous system as it carries these "instructions." That the heart is represented by Tiphareth, the center of harmony and beauty on the Tree, indicates that it is the most important organ in the body. The heart chakra conveys its prana to that center within mankind so that he may be stimulated to acquire and develop its principle of magnanimity, selflessness, and love. The endocrine gland into which this prana is received is the thymus, which, as discussed previously, is responsible for the body's immunity. The thymus also works with the adrenals in dealing with stressful situations.

The fifth chakra is the throat, or laryngeal, chakra, and like the splenic chakra, it circumscribes the intersection of paths joining vertical and horizontal principles. The horizontal principles are Chesed and Geburah, while the vertical principles of will are represented by Daath and Tiphareth. The throat chakra, although expressing itself in and through mankind, directly relates to man as he responds to Divine thought and, in turn, expresses that thought through his "spoken word" of creativity. The endocrine gland into which the energy of the throat chakra is directed is the thyroid. Embedded within the thyroid are the parathyroids, represented by Chesed and Geburah, which aid in the thyroid's main function of integrating the intellectual efforts and desires within the structure of metabolism. The thyroid affects both the nerves and the rate of metabolism and is very important in the structure of form. The parathyroids are the gateway to the body's own realization. They govern the bone marrow, as well as control calcium and salts within the blood.

The sixth chakra is the brow, or frontal, chakra; like the fifth chakra, it does not relate as directly to the body of mankind as it does to Divine influence as it flows through man into mankind. The brow chakra has long been known as the "third eye." When fully developed, it vitalizes the aspect known as "clairgnosis," or clear knowing. The endocrine gland energized by the brow chakra is the pituitary, which governs the entire endocrine chain and regulates reproduction and growth. Represented by Daath of Yetzirah, the pituitary is receptive to the force of the pineal gland of the crown chakra. It causes contraction of the smooth muscles, and influences water metabolism.

The seventh chakra is the crown chakra, which energizes the pineal gland. The pineal gland utilizes the thalamus and medulla oblongata in its work of maintaining continuity of consciousness. The pineal gland is considered to be atrophied, but it would be better to say it has yet to be developed. Its purpose via the crown chakra is to bring the pure force of the monad, the Divine spark within man, into mankind's experience. However,

145

man has not yet developed the consciousness strong enough to contain and express this powerful force of will. Esoterically, the pineal gland is considered the gateway to the monad—the Divine spark—because it is able to receive direct influence from Kether, the Crown, of its World. Arising from the juncture of two paths, the crown chakra is a powerful vortex of energy. The thalamus, represented by Binah, is the site from which the optic nerve springs forth within the brain, giving mankind the ability to see. The medulla oblongata, represented by Chokmah, regulates body processes, while protecting and guarding against overstimulation. It is known that nerve impulses occur in the pineal gland in response to light; therefore, it should follow that when the pineal gland is developed, man will be able to receive the pure light aspect of his being.

In addition to their work of absorbing and distributing prana, the chakras interact with the force of kundalini. The effect of kundalini on the chakras results in what are called the "psychic senses." Kundalini, lying at the base of the spine, is a reservoir in which Divinity's will for form is contained; it is used in accordance with the development of man's capability of expressing the principles that it energizes. The growth process itself draws this force into higher levels of consciousness; it never needs to be stimulated in any other way. The stimulation of this force without the proper containment for it results in disaster. It is like opening the floodgates of a dam without having constructed proper channels for the water.

Many individuals have already undergone the awakening of the psychic senses in their evolutionary life span and have now moved beyond their appropriate level, reaching instead for the heart center of Tiphareth. In response to those levels higher than itself, Tiphareth formulates clairgnosis.

It is important for the professional Kabalistic healer to understand the impact of man's mind upon mankind by directives issued through the chakras. A lack of the pranic force, as well as a distortion of the patterns of that force, will evidence itself in the physical or emotional level of mankind. The understanding of the chakral influence requires an in-depth study that results in a thorough knowledge of the principles of the Tree, an understanding of expression of these principles, and, especially, the intuitive knowing (clairgnosis) of just where each individual stands in relationship to the chakral influence. This simple clarification and description has been given in order to explain that there is a type of transmission of directives issued from the mind of man, and even from levels higher than that, that extend to mankind through aspects of man's consciousness. Just as the higher levels impact the lower, what occurs on the lower has ramifications on the higher. Thus, the Kabalistic healer must look at all aspects of life from physical activity to the higher levels of consciousness in order to ascertain the origin of the disharmony.

147

17

In His Image,
Man Creates Mankind

Just as man is created in the image and likeness of God,
mankind is created in the image and likeness of man. During
gestation, a baby is instilled with the same potential as its parents. However, a baby creates its body based upon the needs of
its own consciousness. Although man contains his innate Divine
potential, in Kabalistic terms known as the Adam Kadmon, he
creates his vehicle or body in accordance with a pattern of consciousness drawn from his own experience as a mind-being. This
pattern is formulated by the totality of man's consciousness existing within the World of Yetzirah, the world of the mind. The
actual body is, in a sense, a dimensional symbol reflected by that
pattern, a symbol represented by the sensate/physical World of
Assiah. The aspects of the pattern for mankind in Yetzirah will
reflect themselves into the emotional/physical body in Assiah.

Thus a distortion or disease in the physical body reflects the principles and levels within the pattern of the higher world upon which it was built. By placing mankind's body upon the Tree of Life, one can determine which principles and Sephiroth correspond to the levels and aspects of the physical body.

Figure 17.1 illustrates the four planes or major levels of man's expression and the aspects of mankind that relate to those levels. Remember that this diagram is only a generalization. Only individual spiritual counseling by a trained Kabalistic healer can help one to realize how the principles relate to one personally. There are also diseases, as mentioned previously, that are termed general or regional, affecting many parts of the body. Often these are the result of intensified minor disorders accumulated from one's greater span of evolutionary life. Examples of such diseases are cancer, diabetes, epilepsy, hepatitis, leukemia, muscular dystrophy, and rheumatism. If any of these affect one level or aspect more than others, then it is important to take note of the area of intensification.

There are a number of excellent books that describe most diseases in relationship to their causes. But remember, these descriptions are generalizations that must always be further clarified with regard to each individual. For example, cancer usually indicates intolerance or crystallization; diabetes indicates a bitterness regarding one or more aspects of one's life; epilepsy indicates a feeling of persecution, a desire to evade life; hepatitis as it affects the liver relates to anger, rage, or highly charged emotionalism; leukemia indicates a sense of futility, a lack of joy; muscular dystrophy relates to the desire for control; and rheumatism relates to a sense of being victimized, of being used.

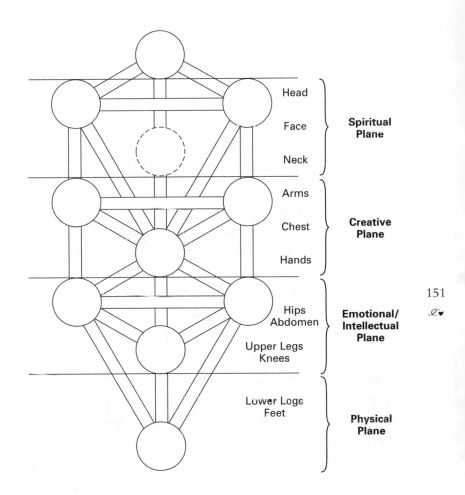

Head

Face **Spiritual Plane**

Neck

Arms

Chest **Creative Plane**

Hands

151

𝒵♥

Hips
Abdomen **Emotional/ Intellectual Plane**

Upper Legs
Knees

Lower Legs
Feet **Physical Plane**

FIGURE 17.1. MAN'S IMAGE OF MANKIND

But remember that it is only because of man's identification with his sensate/material world that his creative ability's consciousness is dominated by it. This changes the innate pattern of balance and harmony into a distorted pattern that produces distortions in the body. One cannot replace those distorted patterns until he establishes the correct replacement. To do this requires effort and responsibility.

Diseases associated with the head, face, and neck are reflections of distortions from the spiritual level and are based on the principles of devotion, receptivity, and detachment. These generally relate to man's innate Divine authority over his life in accordance with that authority's purpose in the incarnated pattern. We are free only when we allow Divine life-will to flow into a pattern appropriate for that flow's expression. Depending on an individual's level of growth, disturbances in these areas can also relate to authority issues with other individuals. For example, diseases or distortions affecting the neck relate to inflexibility, a refusal to accept authority, and a resistance to growth; sinus problems or colds relate to a resistance to establish one's authority, or irritation caused by a situation or person; and afflictions of the throat indicate the inability or reluctance to speak up for oneself.

Creative-level distortions or diseases are associated with one's creativity and mental concepts. They affect such areas as the shoulders, arms, hands, and chest. Such distortions can be present in the back, indicating a lack of support. Distortions in the lower back show a lack of support in physical existence, such as finances or work; those in the middle back suggest a feeling of not being worthy of support; and those in the upper back indicate a lack of emotional support from others. Other creative-level distortions or diseases occur in the heart, relating to creative will, self-worth, self-recognition, and self-nurturing.

Distortions or diseases relating to both the intellectual/ emotional and physical levels affect the hips, abdomen, and knees (intellectual/emotional level) and the lower legs and feet (physical level). For instance, intestinal problems may indicate an improper assimilation of understanding, or not letting go of what is no longer needed. Kidney problems relate to failure and disappointment. The feet represent the foundation upon which one stands, present understanding, and the ability to move forward, while the ankles represent mobility and direction.

Let us look at an example of someone who has chronic lower back pain. Since the back relates to the creative level, this pain indicates that the condition arises from a creative act wherein the individual feels that he has no physical or financial support (lower back). If the individual invests all of his time into starting a business and feels sorry for himself because nobody else has offered time or money, he may come to believe that he is carrying a greater financial and physical burden than he can bear. Eventually this belief, if continued, may cause his condition to worsen—into a slipped disc, for example—until he literally becomes unable to move. Physical accidents also often worsen a condition.

153

One must understand, however, that addressing these distortions is not as simple as merely looking at a chart and diagnosing the source of the problem. Diagnosing the source requires consulting with each individual and understanding his life pattern's expression as well as understanding where that individual stands in spiritual growth.

It is also important to understand that an individual with knee problems is not necessarily lower on the spiritual growth scale than someone who has sinus problems. Growth occurs on a spiral; thus, the individual with knee problems may actually be in a higher cycle than someone with sinus problems. This is similar to the fact that basic subjects are learned in first grade and then repeated, but on a higher level, in second, third, and fourth grades, and so on.

Hippocrates once said, "It is more important to know what kind of person has the disease than what kind of disease the person has." Furthermore, what kind of disease the person has usually indicates what is lacking or distorted within man's pattern for mankind. Disease is a symptom of the distortion, and indicates either an inappropriate application of the principles inherent in man or a need to integrate a certain principle. The disease itself shows where the establishment of balance needs to occur, and if not heeded, its intensity will increase in proportion to the individual's inability or refusal to hear its message.

18

The Healer

When an individual proclaims himself to be a healer, perhaps demonstrating successfully his capabilities, there are many who stand in awe. This emotional force is then directed back to the healer, and unless the healer is balanced and selfless, it can effect a self-image of grandeur. What is interesting about this cycling of life-force energy from those who direct it to the healer is that it can indeed enable the healer to direct even more life-force energy to others. Because this energy makes those receiving it "feel better," even more awe and admiration are directed to the healer. Anytime life-force energy, regardless of its origin, passes through the emotional/intellectual or astral level of the healer, there is the chance that it might empower the ego of the healer. Think of how you feel when someone praises or compliments you. The only way in which the healer's ego is not stimulated by the cycling of energy is when the healer is in balance and detached from ego influence during the healing session. Oftentimes an imbalanced status stimulates both the healer and healee, resulting in a codependency.

Within the esoteric/metaphysical world, healing has become big business—a multitude of books, classes, tools, and other related services for healing are available. Some of these are effective, others accomplish little, and a few can be very detrimental if one is not aware of just what occurs in the transmission of energy. Both secular and esoteric/metaphysical healing methods can indeed be of great help in the establishment of body wholeness, but they are just that: a help. They are the means to an end, not the goal.

You would not want someone whose medical expertise comes only from *Gray's Anatomy,* or even someone in his first year of medical school, to perform heart or brain surgery on you. If such surgery were indicated, you would seek out a professional who possesses the proper credentials attesting to his capability as a surgeon. The medical field has established rules and regulations regarding one's acquiring the title of physician; significantly, however, there is no governing body that determines who is effective at issuing prescriptions for and manipulating and/or directing healing energies. These energies are intangible, because they cannot be physically seen, but it would be very foolish to deny their existence or potency. X rays cannot be seen with the naked eye, and yet look at their potency. Think of energies even more powerful than X rays being used by those who have little or no training or those who have set themselves up as experts without even realizing or caring about the impact and devastation that can be caused by the inappropriate use of such energies. Many assume themselves to be accredited healers, dispensing spiritual healing energies, and some, exploiting the feelings of others for fulfillment of their own self-importance and greed, actually prevent an individual from successfully completing his life pattern.

There are those who, through study, learn to express their innate healing ability, and who have, through a process of self-development, established the balance and strength through which that ability can serve others. Just as one is discerning about his physician, he should be as discerning, if not more so, in his selection of a spiritual healer. The purpose of the healer is to empower the individual to establish his own wholeness. We must remember that each individual has the potential to heal himself, yet often that capability cannot be expressed. To understand the proper role of the healer, imagine jump-starting someone's automobile—you have to disconnect the jumper cables before he can drive away. Your help has been crucial, but now his car has to generate its own power.

Most spiritual healers, regardless of the manner in which they work or what terms they use to identify their particular processes and manner of healing, bring forth the life-force of Netzach of Yetzirah as it is empowered by collective or universal life-force of Chesed, through their unconscious minds. What distinguishes spiritual healers from each other is their ability to center themselves and establish a clear channel through the unconscious mind for the conveyance of this powerful life-force energy. This does not mean that the healer may not have problems of his own, but that he is able to set them aside while he is transmitting healing energy. Never allow yourself to receive healing energy from someone who is obviously emotionally distraught or whose diagnosis of your distortion or disease is based on "textbook" definitions. The best physician is one who listens to his patient, knowing that each individual is unique even when displaying similar symptoms.

The Kabalistic healer acknowledges the importance of all levels of healing—physical, emotional, and creative. His purpose is to work in conjunction with, not in opposition to, physical and emotional healing. Kabalistic healing is directed to the source of the distortion yet also acknowledges the need for additional professional help as needed on those levels reached by the distortion that do not relate to his expertise.

158

The road to becoming a Kabalistic healer is a long one, the first part of which is devoted exclusively to self-development. This self-development includes integration to the highest degree possible of these principles of man, since the healer cannot direct to others what he does not himself have. The journey involves self-analysis, self-motivation, and self-direction as one evolves toward Self-consciousness, or superconsciousness. This journey requires years of study and growth. The development of Self-consciousness also includes the development of clairgnosis, a result of that growth process. Clairgnosis is not intuition; rather, intuition is the expression, or appropriate application, of clear knowing.

Kabalistic healing involves a state of becoming and can be expressed through whatever vocation the individual is involved in. In fact, because Kabalistic healing extends from the superconscious level of the soul, we can say that it often has a life of its own, being projected by the soul to others even when it is not actively practiced. When one becomes the Tree of Life in totality, one does not need to consciously project its principles where they are needed, since the core or heart of that Tree is the soul. The techniques taught in Kabalistic healing are modified to suit the particular healing expression of the individual. For instance, a therapist conveys healing through the counseling process, a chiropractor through adjustments to the body, and a spiritual counselor through a soul-to-soul connection. Those who follow the vocation called Kabalistic healing, however, are experienced spiritual counselors who apply a technique of healing energy transfer. As part of their counseling, they refer an individual to a therapist when emotional disturbances indicate the need for therapy, or to a chiropractor when it is evident that body adjustments must be made. The Kabalistic healer also directs one for medical advice and treatment as needed, since the physical body itself often needs the aid of a physician to establish balance. For example, while spiritual counseling and healing energies are used with one who has diabetes, perhaps to reveal the source of the bitterness within the concepts of the pattern creating that disorder, it is also vitally important to continue treating the physical body as indicated by the disease.

Each level—physical, emotional, and creative—has its professionals, and to achieve wholeness within man/mankind, it is important for the professionals on each level to acknowledge and work in harmony with those on other levels. The physician or chiropracter uses his knowledge to empower the body to heal itself; the therapist uses his knowledge to empower the revelation and correction of unconscious reactive patterns; and the

Kabalistic healer uses his knowledge for the empowerment of those Divine principles within each individual. This last knowledge is one of consciousness, not intellect; it allows the level of the Self—to whatever degree it is developed in the healer—to impress its harmony and principles upon that same level within the individual seeking healing.

Distortions or diseases occurring on the physical and emotional levels have their origins within man and are brought into existence through his creative ability, based on the patterns he holds for the expression of the principles of his existence and whether these principles are in balance or distorted. When the Self or superconscious within each individual is developed, man will then respond to what is called the "perfect pattern" emanated by Divine life-will and create that pattern into mankind's existence. To develop the Self requires an educational growth process revealing which principles are yet to be developed or which principles are distorted. One way that distorted or undeveloped principles are indicated is by disease. God created man, which is not a singular individual but a group consciousness composed of the many sparks of Divine life contained in that collective mind or soul. Thus it is upon the collective level that the greatest impact is made on each individual spark, and it is to this level that the Kabalistic healer is able to raise his consciousness during the healing and counseling process. To do this requires a developmental/transformative process such as that of Kabalah.

19

Healing

The word *heal* is derived from the Old English word *hal,* meaning "whole." Webster's defines the word *heal* as "to make sound or whole; to restore to health; to cause to be overcome." Businesses related to health and healing number in the thousands. The amount of money spent by individuals attempting to achieve and maintain physical and emotional health is mind-boggling. There are few people, if any, in this world who have not sought healing in some manner. Relief from physical and emotional distortions enables one to live a life of greater ease, and so much effort is expended to prevent such disturbances. However, as stated previously, man must begin to investigate the source or root of the disturbances, for just as pruning a tree causes its branches to grow back even stronger, disturbances will keep coming back unless they are eliminated entirely.

It is important to understand that the physician does not heal the body. He corrects, either by medication or manipulation, a structural imbalance, which then allows life-force to maintain the body's existence. For instance, if one breaks an arm, a physician encloses it in a cast, immobilizing the arm until the body's healing process reunites the broken pieces of bone. The body itself accomplishes the healing, while it is the job of the physician to establish the right circumstances in which that healing can occur. Oftentimes a certain medication or surgery is indicated. Insulin is given to a diabetic whose pancreas no longer produces it, and this enables the body to continue the process of life. The proper dose of insulin is most important, since too little or too much could result in death. Therefore, the knowledge of the correct dose—as well as of the fact that it was the absence of insulin that caused the body to malfunction—is provided by the physician healer. He knows that a certain element necessary for the body's functioning is missing. This same theory applies to all levels of healing, but in the ultimate sense only the individual, using what has been prescribed for each and all levels applicable for healing, can establish his own wholeness.

Regardless of the terminology used, all healing energies are brought into existence through the levels of the mind represented by the Sephiroth on the middle pillar of the Tree of Life. However, there is a duality of force and form energies that relates to each stage of the mind's intent. And in relationship to evolutionary growth, each stage is more empowered and refined than the previous one. Contrary to popular belief, the world's oldest profession is that of the healer. Since its origin, mankind has continuously sought ways to relieve pain and disease. These ways have related to each stage of consciousness through which mankind evolved. As mankind became more complex in his expression, the methods and types of healing increased; today, there are a multitude of books, classes, schools, and teachers of healing techniques. Regardless of technique, however, the same basic principles or energies are used. The flow of all types of healing energies can be depicted upon the Tree of Life.

There are only three aspects of the mind (superconscious, unconscious, and conscious) through which life-force is directed, as well as all of the principles represented by the Sephiroth upon the Tree. One of these aspects, the unconscious, has a vertical duality, which means that, depending on the level of the healer's consciousness, the unconscious can be impressed by the super-conscious mind or soul. All levels of healing are latent in each individual; however, people called "healers" are those who through study, personal development, and a desire to help others have opened their consciousnesses to receive and direct healing energies from the universal "reservoir." In the case of Kabalistic healing, development of the Tree of Life within oneself—that Tree being universal—enables one to direct its principles to others. The Kabalistic healer must be able to achieve a state of balance. The closer in awareness he is in consciousness to Tiphareth on the Tree, the more able he will be to invoke and direct the energies of the entire Tree.

Figure 19.1 depicts the Yetziratic Tree of man and indicates the flow of healing energies as they are directed into form. In looking at the Tree you can see that the life-force energy flows down the right pillar, from Chokmah through Chesed and into Netzach. Life-form, or patterns, flow from Binah to Geburah

163

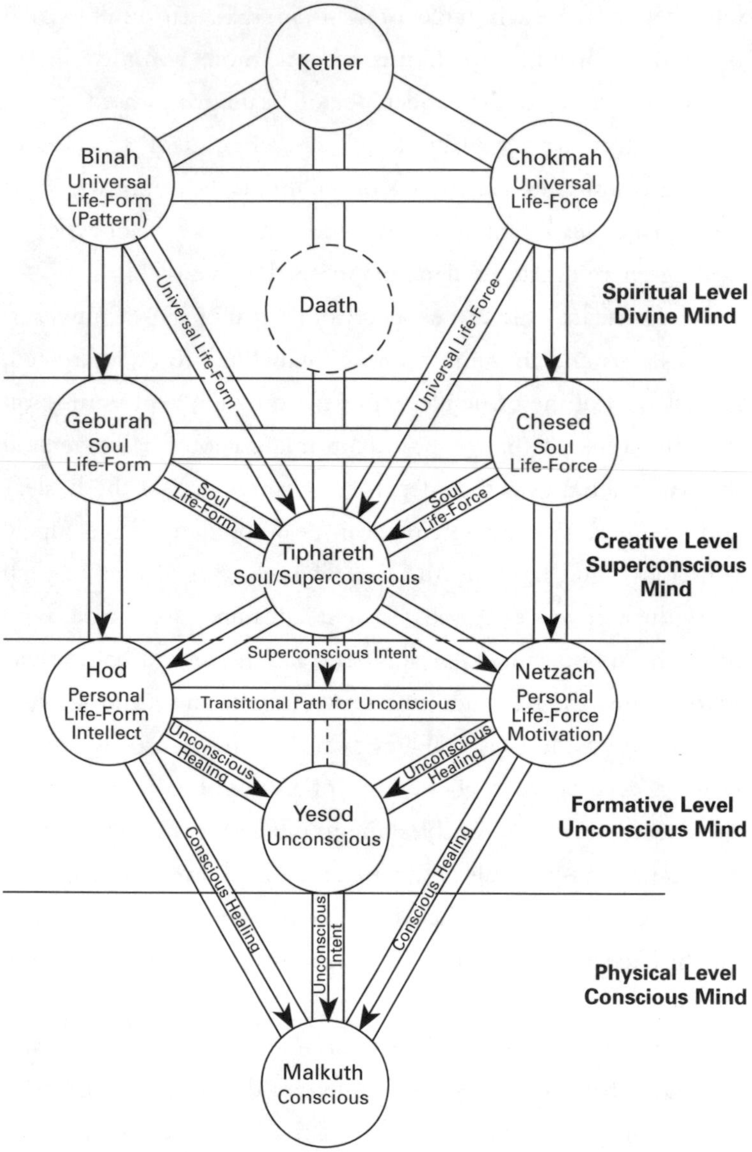

FIGURE 19.1. LEVELS OF HEALING

and into Hod. The life-will or intent that directs force and form descends from Kether to Tiphareth to Yesod and into Malkuth. There is a difference between when the Sephiroth of intent direct the side pillar Sephiroth and when the Sephiroth of intent bring the side pillar energies together into the particular level of intent. One sets the energies into motion down the side pillars, and the other brings them into the middle pillar, creating a balanced union wherein the energies are then expressed by and through the middle pillar. Either way will bring about results; however, middle-pillar expression of intent always ensures that the principles are in balance with each other and directed by the highest level of consciousness the healer is able to achieve.

Let us examine the function of healing as it relates to the lowest level of activity, the conscious mind. This type of healing as it relates to the life experience can be simply illustrated by the example of one who inadvertently cuts himself. His brain, a tool that is empowered by motivation and intellect, would instruct him to bandage and/or medicate the wound so that the body could effectively institute its own healing process. If the wound were severe, the individual would seek the services of a physician, who—through the use of his own brain, motivation, and intellect—would perhaps stitch the wound and inject the individual with antibiotics to prevent infection.

Now let us examine the same use of the conscious mind by a healer who uses the more subtle principles of Netzach and Hod as they relate to creative power and creative ideation. To facilitate the healing of the wound just described, the individual might seek the services of a healer. In a laying-on-of-hands function of healing, the healer, through conscious intent, uses his personal life-force principle to draw upon additional life-force in the application of those energies to the wound, either to alleviate the pain or to accelerate the healing process. The additional life-force is needed to reinstate the balance of that part of the body that has become imbalanced from injury. In this example the force pillar of the Tree is used; however, we can expand it to include the form pillar.

In this case, let us say that the wound occurred due to an emotional outburst of anger, so now we go beyond the healing function relative to the wound itself to the pattern of anger behind it. To deal with his anger, the individual seeks counseling—which, in a sense, the accident was endeavoring to show was needed. The therapist or counselor, through the use of his conscious mind, draws upon the principle of life-form or truth of Hod, investigates the pattern that prompted the anger, and attempts through a correction of that pattern to alleviate the problem. Unless the therapist is a healer and unless the healer is a therapist, one-sided principles are used in an attempt to help the individual reach a balanced state.

The majority of healing techniques today involve the principles of Netzach and Hod, as they are directed through Yesod, the unconscious mind of the healer. Because it exists upon the formative level, which is higher than the conscious mind's physical level, the unconscious is able to use the creative ideation and creative power principles of Netzach and Hod. This type of healing can be impacted by the superconscious mind of Tiphareth if the healer's consciousness can be raised above the path that joins Netzach and Hod. There are times when those who are involved strictly in physical healing of the body, such as doctors and nurses, actually do bring down a higher aspect of healing and guidance from the superconscious mind while not even being aware of it. These individuals usually become quite adept in their fields, they often know even before examination just where within the body the problem lies, and they are able to convey to their patients tremendous confidence and motivation.

The use of visualization in any healing technique restricts the directive force or intent to the formative level. Whether symbolic or explicit, what is visualized uses the principle of Hod, creative ideation, for its formulation within the parameters of the unconscious mind of the healer. These parameters, however, are reactive, not descriptive. The healing energy of life-force, the principle of Netzach, empowers the ideation along with using it as a directive for the flow of healing energy. This flow can either move downward directly into the physical form of the individual seeking healing or can be projected to that same aspect of unconscious mind within that individual, depending upon the system and technique being used. It is important, then, that the unconscious mind of the healer be stabilized in balance and detached from all reactive emotions or feelings during the healing process.

If the consciousness of the healer can be raised above the path that joins Netzach and Hod, the soul or superconscious may be able to direct the principles of Netzach and Hod, which are then drawn to the unconscious of the healer to be further directed into the healing process. Remember that the middle pillar of the Tree expresses only the life-will/intent that either directs the principles of the side pillars or draws those principles to itself upon the various levels of its intent. If there are distorted or imbalanced concepts within the unconscious mind, then the

167

side principles that are drawn to that mind will be affected accordingly, either distorting or diminishing the principles necessary for wholeness, balance, or healing.

The majority of mankind allows the principles of motivation (desire) and intellect to direct their will for action, rather than directing those principles by the will for action. This results in the confusion, chaos, and distortion we see in the world. When centered in the highest level of will possible in accordance with the evolutionary pattern for all man, one is free to use the principles of motivation and intellect rather than be dominated by them. If dominated by them, healing energies may be distorted in accordance with the imbalance within the unconscious mind caused by that domination. This is not to say that a healer is continually in balance, but that he is able to establish that balance when directing healing energies.

The Kabalistic healer has, through a transformative process, developed the state whereby he is able to raise his consciousness to the level of Tiphareth during the healing technique. As the heart or hub of the Tree, Tiphareth is able to direct all of its principles to whatever degree is needed to effect a healing directed by the soul of the individual seeking healing. Tiphareth can draw upon the soul's principles of power and ideation form, Chesed and Geburah, redirecting them through soul intent into the personal power and ideation of the one seeking healing. Tiphareth is also able to draw upon the universal life-force patterns, impressing them upon their lower-level counterparts in accordance with each individual pattern and status. The technique for Kabalistic healing at this level is vastly different from those of the lower levels, but this is not to say that the others are not viable, for even what we call Kabalistic healing uses all levels.

The types of Kabalistic healing are discussed next; they range from over-the-counter, self-prescribed applications, to applications that require a greater understanding of the makeup of man's psyche, to applications that require a process of development similar to that experienced by an aspiring physician. In a sense, Kabalistic healers could be called "soul physicians."

169

20

Conscious
Kabalistic Healing

Without being aware of it, many of us already use self-prescribed Kabalistic healing principles. Much like over-the-counter medications, application of these principles on the conscious and physical level can aid in alleviating distress while enhancing the healing process, especially when one is aware of those principles and their proper application. This is similar to being able to determine whether one needs an aspirin or an antacid.

A variety of interchangeable terms are used to describe the frequencies of the principles represented by the Sephiroth on the Tree of Life. For instance, Tiphareth is the sixth Center or Sephirah and is represented by the number 6 and the sun. It is also known as Ray Six, the soul, superconsciousness, and the Christ Consciousness. But one of its most important attributes is its color, golden yellow, because this color impresses its frequency upon the unconscious mind.

God, as Kether of the Tree of Life, is light, and because God is also everything, this makes the various aspects or principles of God the refraction of light into colors. Therefore, color itself is energy. We can see that energy in its manifestation of the visible electromagnetic spectrum. Because energy exists on all levels, so does color. Our thoughts are projected in color; all healing energy refracts into color. We are unable to see some colors with the naked eye, such as infrared and ultraviolet. Even within the visible spectrum color perception varies. The first words spoken in the Old Testament are "Let there be light . . ." (Genesis 1:3). That God spoke these words indicates the importance of light and its refracted colors.

The level upon which color frequencies are used is particularly relevant. Some years back the *New York Times* ran an article titled "Plain Old Red Light Used to Cure Cancer." The article stated that researchers had noted improvement in cancerous areas that had been showered with red light. This physical application of the red frequency would energize the body's ability to destroy cancer cells, but the respite would probably be short-lived unless the pattern upon which the disease was based was corrected. There is nothing wrong with the respite, but during that time one must devote effort to correct the distorted pattern.

The future will bring increased use of subtle energies such as color and sound in healing and counseling. Color and sound are interchangeable because both define certain energies. Perhaps one day we will see sound and hear color. The parameters of sight and hearing will also widen as mankind's need for expression grows, necessitating a greater area for experience. Color and sound could then become a part of what is termed "vibrational medicine." There are some physicians who practice the most basic type of vibrational medicine: simply by speaking to their patients, they are able to instill feelings of confidence, calmness, and hope. Such physicians are said to have "a good bedside manner." This "manner" is comprised of a vibratory sound that contains and projects the physician's compassion, leadership, and guidance.

For some time it has been accepted that color is important; however, its associations, use, and interpretations have been many and varied. Randomly select five books on color and you will find at least four different opinions. Most Kabalistic writers use and define color as it was brought forward from the ancient tradition, and nearly all are in agreement. A great deal of understanding of subtle color frequencies can be gained through the study of the color archetypes of the Tree of Life. The frequency is the same whether the color is expressed in pigment or light, and a combination of colors represents a combination of the principles that each color represents.

Just as with over-the-counter medications, it is important to know both the proper principle and its proper dosage. But since color is used in daily living, simple common sense is required in its application. One should be able to choose clothes of appropriate colors to benefit the personal experiences of that day. For example, if mental focus is needed, wearing medium blue would enhance that clarity. In a stressful situation, green or yellow would be appropriate. Similarly, painting certain areas to suit their functions enhances their use. Because these are only generalizations, they do not require concern regarding the proper amounts or doses. On the other hand, continued application of color to a specific area does warrant such concern. One would not continue to apply an antibiotic ointment to a wound after it has healed, nor would one overdose on aspirin or antacids.

The following is a brief description of the attributes of the colors that represent the principles of the Sephiroth of the Tree of Life as depicted in figure 20.1. These colors can help effect balance within the existence of mankind. The colors representing the Sephiroth in the World of Briah are used because they represent man's highest potential of expression. To attain that for which man strives, he must use the principles of perfection found in that attainment. These principles make up what is termed the Adam Kadmon, the image of God that man is to become.

Kether: Pure White Brilliance. White light is the total combination of all colors, and it refracts into the rainbow spectrum. White pigment reflects all colors, absorbing none. White is the frequency of coagulation, the condensing of force into form. Interestingly, white is the common color of bandages. White is also the traditional color for marriage, the union of force and form.

Chokmah: Silver. Chokmah is depicted as gray on many Trees. Its silver hue is not actually a color but an attempt to portray a metaphysical frequency. Silver is pure spiritual force and promotes devotion and high ideals. It should not be used or worn in large amounts, for its impact could be too intense, prompting Chokmah's vice of misused power.

Binah: Indigo. Black is most often used to portray this color; however, Binah's frequency is much higher than black. Indigo represents the concealment of light, protection from the blinding brilliance of Divinity, releasing only as much as one is able

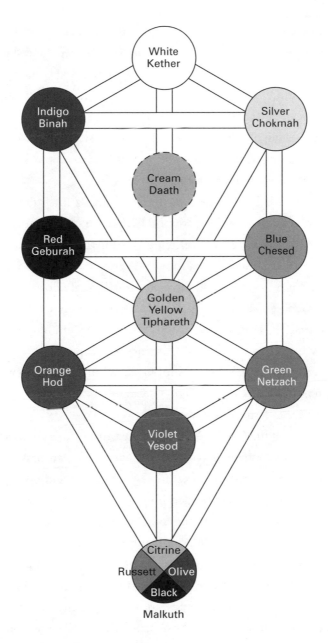

FIGURE 20.1. PRINCIPLES OF THE TREE OF LIFE IN COLOR

to withstand at any given time. Indigo has often been related to the color of the night sky, and is defined as being a deep violet-blue. It is a color of concealment, receptivity, restriction, and containment.

Daath: Cream. Cream is the frequency of sensitivity, vision, realization, and responsiveness. It is excellent for meditation areas, but might promote too much sensitivity in larger areas. When wearing cream clothing, it is best to combine it with another complementary color.

Chesed: Blue. Blue, a primary color, is a force frequency, stepped down from the silver of Chokmah. Rather than the intense impact force of silver, blue is a binding force that both promotes and contains expansion. It is a mental color of inspiration and inventiveness, and facilitates intellectual effort or study.

Geburah: Red. Red is another primary color and represents strength, vitality, and passion. It is an excellent frequency to wear when energy is needed, but since it can promote nervousness, temper, and passion, it should be worn with a grounding frequency. Red is often used in restaurants and bars, since it increases the desire to eat and drink.

Tiphareth: Golden Yellow. As the third primary color, yellow is a creative frequency and is excellent to wear or surround oneself with. It produces cheerfulness, creativity, and courage. It is a balance color and its golden hue takes that frequency into the spiritual virtues of thoughtfulness, unselfishness, and dedication.

Netzach: Green. Green, a combination of blue and yellow, is the first of the secondary colors to be encountered in the descent of the Tree. All of the personal frequencies lower than Tiphareth contain its frequency, thus instilling the intent of the soul or superconscious into those principles of its expression into activity. Green is the color of emotional strength, inner fortitude, and reserve energy. Because green is a healing force, it is excellent in any type of healing work. It is one of the most restful colors of the spectrum. It is not as compatible as yellow or blue with a study environment, since it may not be stimulating enough for mental work; but once the mental aspect has been acquired, this frequency can be the motivational power for it.

Hod: Orange. Another secondary color, combining the strength and energy of Geburah with the creativity, courage, and selflessness of Tiphareth, orange is a frequency of communication. It promotes a desire to share ideas and thoughts, and gives one a feeling of optimism and self-confidence. It is an excellent color to wear in a situation where communication is essential.

Yesod: Violet. This frequency, though on the middle pillar of the Tree, is often not an easy color to wear, since, by its very nature, it attempts to align one with his pattern as impacted by the intent of the soul. This color can produce a yearning or uneasy mind, which can be beneficial because it promotes movement and growth. Violet is the color of talent seeking an outlet in material expression, and it conveys a sensitivity to beauty in all areas.

Malkuth: Citrine, Olive, Russet, and Black. Citrine (greenish yellow) is the frequency of spiritual perception, broadmindedness, and tolerance. It drives one onward for the betterment of humanity and the establishment of balance in the world. It is the citrine quadrant of Malkuth into which the final paths of the Tree flow, indicating that the final expression of all of the Divine principles is for the evolution of mankind.

Olive is the frequency of dissolution and has long been associated with mankind's concept of death. Despite its appeal,

177

one should not wear olive in large amounts unless he has disassociated with the concept of death as loss and has come to understand that death is necessary for dissolution so that something new can be formed.

Russet, a balancing, stabilizing frequency, represents a foundation gained from past experience. It holds whatever is grounding within until it is needed. Esoterically, it is considered the frequency of all that is not self and conveys a sense of well-being and security.

Black, like white, is not really a color. White is a frequency of form, while black is a frequency of movement, for it warns or draws attention to something. It arrests and outlines what is to be noticed. It is the frequency of cancellation and the absence of color, absorbing all the refractions of light. Black is the color related to funerals, the cancellation of life in a certain form. Black is the common color of printing, for it draws attention to the words.

The shade or tone of a color relates to the level of its expression: the darker the shade the more physical the expression, the lighter the more spiritual; with many gradations in between. For instance, a very light green indicates spiritual strength and fortitude, a slightly darker green indicates those aspects relative to the creative level, medium green relates to the emotional/intellectual level, and deep green relates to the physical aspects of strength and fortitude.

For a more thorough description of these principles, one can look to the astrological definitions of the planets that represent the Sephiroth, given in chapter 8. Use color in your life by consciously surrounding yourself with or wearing colors that complement your daily activities or enhance the development of

178

those aspects of the psyche that are indicated in your life. This is a simple but effective way to identify with those principles that make up the being we call man. They are not cure-alls any more than an aspirin will cure a brain tumor that is causing a headache, yet aspirin can alleviate the pain, allowing the individual the freedom of activity by which he may seek a cure for the brain tumor. Just as anyone can use an aspirin, anyone can become aware of the principles of the Tree of Life as they are translated in the frequencies of colors. This awareness helps establish the identification of oneself within the unconscious as a mind-being comprised of those same refractions of Divine light.

Be aware of the colors surrounding you in your world. The blue sky is the essence of expansion and freedom, the green of the trees and plants surrounds you with a healing and balancing frequency, and the colors of plants' blooms and fruits present the entire spectrum based on that balance. Take note of which colors you dislike, since they often represent principles that you have been reluctant to integrate. We all prefer certain colors and are more compatible with some frequencies than others, but any strong aversion to a certain color should be investigated.

God is Light, and the children emanated from God are Light. We may come to a greater conscious and unconscious realization of God and ourselves by understanding and using the colors into which God's Light refracted.

21

Unconscious
Kabalistic Healing

Each successively higher level of Kabalistic healing requires
the use of the levels preceding it in order to reach that level.
"Unconscious" does not mean that one is totally unaware of the
process, but that the individual utilizes a level not perceived by
the physical senses. Thus, it is unconscious to him.

Each successive level of the mind is associated with a
higher frequency. The use of a higher frequency is faster and
more efficient than a lower one; however, it also requires consciousness' ability to work within that level. Man's consciousness
is viable within the level of the unconscious mind when he is
dreaming. Visualization techniques of any kind take place upon
the level of the unconscious, and what is visualized cannot be
perceived by the physical senses.

Because the frequency of the unconscious is higher than that of the conscious mind, one must be more careful and selective in using and/or directing energies from its level. For example, a nurse has a greater understanding of medications than the average person, because he must dispense a great many medications in the course of his work.

This chapter presents two methods of directing healing energies that can be used by those who have integrated the principles of the Tree within themselves—not necessarily by studying the Kabalah, but by the process of growth. They do require, however, an understanding of the principles and the color frequencies to which they relate. One must remember that it takes time and patience to develop an efficient and effective use of healing energies. A great concert pianist begins by learning the scales; after that, his ability grows through dedication and practice. In the case of using healing energies, that dedication becomes right motivation. To direct a certain principle to another is similar to suggesting a certain medication to another individual. One becomes fully responsible for the results, and if the medication is not correct, one incurs the consequence.

The first step in utilizing any higher-frequency healing method requires centering one's own awareness. If your feelings are running rampant, then meditate or do whatever is necessary to bring yourself into balance. Although it may require some amount of effort, when utilizing higher healing energies it is imperative to be calm and centered. One might say that you must set "yourself" aside; if you are unable to do this, then any attempt to direct higher healing energies will be futile and produce even greater distortion. Remember that healing energies are just that: energies. When directed to a specific distortion they can either alleviate or worsen it, depending upon the state of the consciousness directing those energies.

Because healing energy is derived from a source termed Divinity, an acknowledgment of some kind of that source should be expressed within the consciousness of the individual healer. The movement of the Spirit of God emanated the creation; therefore man (mind) should develop and retain some realization of that Spirit within himself in order to align with its flow. This is spirituality, not religion. The structure called religion is but a containment for the concepts defining the expression of Spirit into a particular form. The containment is secondary to the realization of that Spirit or Divine life. However, all too often we disagree over the containments, neglecting the reason for their existence. Mankind is dying from thirst while arguing about the design and color of the cup that holds water.

To aid in establishing the realization of your own core of Divine life, you can formulate a prayer to be said before proceeding with directing healing energy. You can also visualize yourself surrounded by light. Those more familiar with esoteric studies can say the Great Invocation, which is an invocation of those middle-pillar principles of the Tree of Life. The method one uses is not as important as establishing the realization of that flow of Divine life-power, which is enhanced by some chosen method of containment.

Chapter 20 discussed the conscious use of colors as they represent the principles of the Tree of Life. This application can be taken to the unconscious level, but doing so requires a greater familiarity with those principles, if only because higher-level

183

"medications" have greater potency than their conscious counterparts. For this technique, which relates to the unconscious
level of visualization, visualize yourself enclosed within a particular color. For instance, if you were studying, visualizing yourself surrounded within the frequency of blue would aid that
process. This would be especially helpful if you were studying in
a room painted green, which is not conducive to mental applications. The effect of this visualization, which itself may take only
a few minutes, lasts much longer, since the time-space point on
the unconscious level expands to a far greater length of time on
the physical level. Depending on circumstances, a few minutes
of color-projection visualization can last for an hour in physical
existence. If one is unable to visualize a certain color, then he
needs only to hold the name of that color in his mind with the
same intent. Thought itself contains and responds to the power
of intent; thus it can be said that energy follows thought. In this
method, one uses conscious directives for unconscious-level
energies. Due to these energies' higher frequencies, this method
requires less time to be effective than that of their physical-color
counterparts. However, to use this level one needs the ability to
formulate its force, center oneself, and raise consciousness to that
level of Yetzirah.

Another application of this first method is to visualize
yourself either within a sphere of golden yellow or, preferably,
within a beautiful golden-yellow temple. This color represents
the principle of Tiphareth; soul or superconsciousness. After
centering your consciousness on this visualization, mentally state
your name or the name of an individual, animal, or situation to
which you wish to direct healing energy. If possible, visualize that

name before you, and, if possible, allow it to be transformed into its image. Surround yourself, or that image for which you are seeking healing, with the most brilliant light you can envision. Simultaneously, mentally direct that light by silently stating the name referring to that image, and attempt to direct that energy to either that same level within yourself or another. Visualize either yourself or the image you have created surrounded by the light, until you feel that there is no longer a transmission occurring. This should take no more than five minutes, with ten minutes being the maximum time needed for this type of transmission. As you let the image fade, or the light surrounding you to dissipate, express your gratitude for the Divine life within you that has allowed this process to occur. For this technique to succeed, your consciousness must remain within the golden-yellow sphere or temple while the healing light is invoked. This light then holds all the refractions or principles that, when directed by the soul, can be applied in the proper amounts and areas as needed. Again, the efficacy of this technique depends on the strength, balance, and awareness of the healer's consciousness.

185

Using a second method of unconscious Kabalistic healing on yet a higher level, but only for yourself, necessitates visualizing the Tree of Life with its Sephiroth in color. It entails the same beginning procedure as the first method; namely, centering yourself and developing a realization, through prayer or knowing, of your own Divine center. Following this, you can again visualize yourself within either a sphere or temple of golden yellow. Once again, see your own name before you, as you petition your soul to bring forth the particular principle that is needed for healing or balance within your life. You then visualize before you the Tree of Life, whose Sephiroth are of the colors and locations described in chapter 20. Only the Sephiroth, not the paths, must be visualized in color. You then ask for the particular principle "prescribed" by the soul to reveal itself. When this is effective, one of the Sephiroth will either increase in size or appear to move from its place upon the Tree toward you. Remain totally receptive. Do not intellectualize anything that happens, or you will draw your consciousness back to the level upon which this technique is not viable. Accept and note the first frequency that draws your attention, letting it surround you for a few minutes. Then, as before, give thanks to the Divine intent within you for presenting to you the aspect that needs strengthening. Afterward, recall that principle; endeavor to bring it into your life for the next few days, a week at most. In meditation you may surround yourself with its frequency, or use it in your daily life as much as possible.

It is important to always remember to express your gratitude for what you have been given. This does not mean that Divinity or the Tree of Life needs your gratitude, but that you, yourself, need the expression of it. It enables you to develop receptivity to that flow of Divine principles, and it aids in the development of your unconscious acceptance and realization of these principles.

These techniques require one's ability to raise consciousness to a higher level of awareness. This is not too difficult for those who are accustomed to the practice of meditation, where Divine intent reaches down as man reaches up. Meditation is essential for those involved in healing practices. It is also important for those who are not, since it is a way for one to bring his consciousness into balance, allowing it to be impacted by the flow of Divine life. Meditation is acknowledged by both physicians and metaphysicians to aid in the relief from stress and to help alleviate many disorders caused by stress, and should thus become an important part of one's daily life.

The second technique is effective to the extent of one's ability to achieve the level of consciousness upon which it becomes viable. Upon that level, however, it is an extremely powerful process that requires faith, hope, and love. Faith, as you know, can move mountains, and all you are requesting is the movement of energy. Hope is the vital state of knowing that all is proceeding according to the soul's plan. Love is the motivation by which this procedure is carried out in the best interest of that soul's growth. When a pattern is restructured from a higher level, the demonstration of its correction must occur within the life experience. This restructuring can effect rapid changes in one's life expression, but it is also associated with experiences that are designed to determine if the new pattern can be adhered to. You can consider this as a test or, better yet, an opportunity. For unless one can demonstrate the corrected pattern, the old one will be reestablished.

187

Because subtle energies are potent, man must achieve the responsibility to use them appropriately. One does not let a three-year-old randomly choose from the multitude of medications in a drugstore that can relieve a cold. He might believe he is old enough to do so, but his inappropriate selection might prove otherwise. Thus it is important for each individual to develop the responsibility, strength, and awareness necessary to direct energies that he knows little about.

22

Superconscious
Kabalistic Healing

The highest level of healing, derived from the soul or super-consciousness, is achieved when the Kabalistic healer uses all levels of healing while remaining centered in consciousness in Tiphareth, the Sephirah of balance and harmony. Kabalistic healing utilizes both the force and form principles of the Tree in a step-by-step direction, culminating in a soul-to-soul transmission of Tiphareth's essence as it directs the other principles of the Tree of Life to the soul level or superconsciousness of another individual.

The Kabalistic healer does not direct his energies downward; rather, he directs a lateral transmission from each level within himself to that same level within the individual receiving the energy. This requires the establishment of the Tree of Life within the healer, acquired through years of spiritual study and growth, which allows him to raise and lower his consciousness as needed when working with another individual and to address all three levels—conscious, unconscious, and superconscious—in the healing process. The two lower levels—the conscious and unconscious—express duality; the superconscious does not. Thus, working from the superconscious level requires a complete reversal of the techniques used for the lower levels.

The Kabalistic healer begins on the conscious level, utilizing spiritual counseling on what we might term the "Jacob's ladder" of healing. At first he tries to help the individual reach an understanding of what his particular distortion or disease is a symptom of. This is important, because the understanding necessary to reform distorted concepts or patterns can be instilled only by the one holding those concepts. The time needed to correct a distortion is directly proportional to the time it took to create it. However, when a higher frequency of energy is applied, it reduces that length of time. The most common element lacking in healing techniques is a form of healing counseling that balances the force of healing energy. Such counseling includes an explanation of disease and pain, and then endeavors to help an individual arrive at an understanding of why his particular disease or pain is occurring. Once this understanding is brought into the conscious mind, the individual can, through this understanding, begin to correct the distortion or integrate the principle indicated. Consequently, there will be no reason for the disease or pain to continue. It is important to understand, however, that it is not simply the conscious mind that must be "convinced" but also the unconscious, and this might require more time than is available during the current lifetime. Although the healer is aware of the causes of distorted patterns that create certain diseases, his responsibility is not to tell or dictate those reasons but to help the individual arrive at his own understanding.

Through meditation and study, the Kabalistic healer develops clairgnosis, or clear knowing, also termed intuition. This enables him to work more effectively, particularly while helping the individual arrive at his own understanding. The Kabalistic healer recognizes the importance of physical and psychological medicine, advising one to obtain such help when the need for it is indicated. Remember that the Kabalistic healer, upon whatever level he addresses an individual, is working from the superconscious level. He must help the "healee" establish receptivity to the energies directed by and through the Tiphareth, or soul level, of the healer to that same level within the recipient, so that the energies may be used in accordance with the intent of the recipient's own superconscious.

The Kabalistic healer provides the vehicle through which energy brought up to the soul level—as well as universal energy brought down to that level—can be transmitted to the recipient. He then provides conscious direction and understanding to facilitate a receptive and balanced state enabling the energies to be received and utilized by the recipient properly and without waste or interruption of the flow. This requires intense personal development along with a thorough understanding of the spiritual nature of man. This personal development includes the growth or establishment of the principles of the Tree, and the personal integration of those principles enables the Kabalistic healer to draw upon their universal counterparts. Many Kabalistic healing systems use an invocation that includes the mental or audible recitation of the Divine names on the middle pillar of the Tree as they represent those principles in the highest World, Atziluth. While techniques may vary, nearly all relate to and use similar expressions of the Tree's energies.

The techniques themselves are quite simple, but developing the strength and state of consciousness whereby they can be effectively used is more complex. It involves much more than merely combining ingredients for a recipe. The whole process depends on the strength of inner development and the ability of the healer to achieve a detached and balanced state while working with another individual.

Just as ethical standards apply to nearly every profession, the same is true for the Kabalistic healer, who, one might say, has the "soul life" of another individual in his hands. This is why caution should be used in the selection of a healer of any type, for a healer who transforms energies through an imbalanced nature will only add to the distortion within another.

The highest level of Kabalistic healing relates to the soul. This requires the ability to center consciousness in the apparent "nothingness" of that level, a level beyond the duality of the lower levels yet much more powerful in the expression of life-will. The ability to raise consciousness to that level and then effect healing from it takes considerable practice. Because that healing derives from a level that does not impact the senses, one has little or no immediate feeling of its impact. The higher the energy transmission, the more subtle the impact of the energy. In this soul-level healing work, the powerful soul or superconscious will within the healer can direct any or all principles or healing essences to that same level within the recipient to be used in accordance with his pattern. It is not that the Kabalistic healer cannot apply the principles he feels are needed by the other individual, but that only the soul of that individual really knows what is appropriate for him.

The Kabalistic healer climbs the Jacob's ladder of healing, working upon each and every level, culminating on the highest level, where the term *soul physician* truly applies. He aligns himself with the Universal Tree of Life and is thus able to invoke the energies or principles of that Tree in a manner indicated by the healee's distortion or disease. The rise in consciousness above the conscious and unconscious minds enables the healer to work in a realm wherein the collective soul of man exists. The application of intent or will to that level allows the energies to be directed without being subjected to any distortions that might bring them down into the lower levels. The force of will of the healer is necessary to propel healing energies from the soul level, yet it is the soul or superconscious itself that directs them. The technique for this type of transmission is quite different from these techniques of visualization or other sub-soul levels of healing. In a sense, it could be said to be the opposite of these techniques, because consciousness is directed up to soul healing rather than healing energies being brought down to the levels of the conscious and unconscious minds.

Tools are available that can enhance the transmission of healing energy. One such tool is the double-terminated healing crystal developed by Marcel Vogel (1917–1991). Marcel Vogel, a scientist at IBM for twenty-seven years, grew up believing in a higher power that could be contacted by prayer and meditation, and he claimed that many of his inventions were the result of the

193

power of prayer. At age eleven, Vogel discovered a synthetic chemical compound that produced a chemiluminescence that matched the light of the firefly. By age fifteen, he was synthesizing for manufacture a number of important phosphors. After selling his business, Vogel Luminescence Corporation, in which he was a pioneer in the manufacture of fluorescents, he went to work for IBM in 1957 as a research scientist, later to become IBM's senior scientist. Over the next twenty-seven years, Vogel did pioneering research in magnetics, opti-electrical devices, and liquid crystal systems, and along with IBM was awarded more than one hundred patents. Among his many inventions was the coating for computer hard disks, still used today in IBM products. Vogel's transformation from rational to spiritual scientist began after he read an article in *Argosy* magazine by Cleve Backster titled "Do Plants Have Emotions?" Vogel began extensive experimentation based on the findings of Backster, the results of which made Vogel a celebrity. But of far greater importance was Vogel's discovery, from a scientific point of view, that thoughts have power and that other kingdoms, such as the plant and mineral kingdoms, are affected by those thoughts.

Vogel's first encounter with the subtle energy potential of quartz crystal occurred in 1974, and after working with crystals, he realized that they could be used to benefit mankind. Deciding to devote the rest of his life to discovering the uses of subtle energies, he retired from IBM in 1984 to establish his own research lab, Psychic Research, Inc., where a tremendous amount of research on the use of crystals was conducted until his death in 1991.

Vogel found limitations in natural crystals. They did not sufficiently cohere to the field that comes from the mind and body of a person. He felt that by cutting and faceting natural quartz, he could amplify the potential information storage capacity. Think of a ruby: A natural ruby is just a nondescript piece of stone, but put it on a faceting machine and you have a gem. Go one step further and take that same ruby, carefully cut it and polish it into a cylinder, put booster windows on it so that light pumped into it is reflected back and forth, and you have a laser.

Since the early 1900s it has been known that quartz is a resonator and amplifier of energy. What was not known, prior to Vogel's research, was that quartz crystal is also capable of amplifying "subtle energies," including thought energy. This had remained difficult to demonstrate because regardless of how fine the quality of the crystal used in a given test was, the conditions under which the crystal formed were idiosyncratic. Simply stated, no two crystals are identical, and in science, a theory cannot be based on a single case. The amplification of thought energy includes so much "static" (other vibrations) that it becomes lost in the noise. Vogel discovered the answer to this problem. He found that when quartz is cut along the c-axis (the line of symmetry within the crystal perpendicular to all other axes) in the shape of the Kabalistic Tree of Life, it resonates to one frequency. It so happens that the frequency, which turned out to be 454, is the same vibratory rate that he measured for water using a psychotronic measuring device called the Omega-5. Since the body is approximately 70 percent water, one can see the impact of this type of energy on the physical body. However, the laserlike healing crystal is also able to amplify and direct thought energies to those higher or subtle levels as well, becoming a valuable tool for the transmission of Kabalistic healing on all levels.

Figure 22.1 depicts the healing crystal cut in the shape of the Tree of Life. In his many workshops, Vogel described how this crystal came into existence: "With unshakable faith, I prayed and meditated for two years and then, one morning I awoke and in my waking state I saw this shape. It appeared as—you might call it a dream or vision. It stood in front of my mind's eye and it remained that way for minutes, not just a fraction of a second. No words, nothing. Just the image. And though I knew nothing about the Kabalah, what I later discovered that I had seen was the Tree of Life."

It is fortunate that Drew Tousley, Vogel's crystal cutter, is today still cutting these unparalleled healing instruments. To use them, however, requires considerable knowledge and practice of the technique for their application. While the use of the crystal is not absolutely essential, it certainly can enhance and augment the healing process.

In summary, the Kabalistic healer is able to direct healing energies upon all levels: conscious, unconscious, and supercon-scious. The higher the level, the greater the empowerment and the amount of understanding needed to use it. The two lower levels bring the higher energies down either for direct transfer-ence or through visualization, while the higher level requires the ability to raise consciousness to the soul level in a technique vastly different from that viable upon the lower levels.

To outline the technique used for the transference of heal-ing energy from the soul level would produce, at best, ineffec-tiveness in directing energies from levels that first need to be developed within the healer. This, unlike the over-the-counter use of medications, requires an educational and developmental

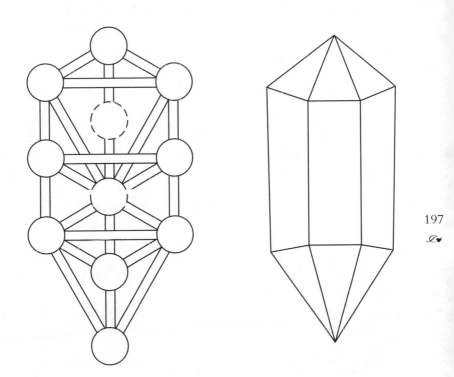

FIGURE 22.1. TREE OF LIFE/VOGEL HEALING CRYSTAL

process under the instruction and guidance of those qualified to present it. A physician must graduate from medical school—a long and arduous process—before he prescribes medications or attempts surgery. Similarly, the Kabalistic healer who directs healing energies from the superconscious or soul level must have completed an educational process relative to that status.

23

The Healee

Although this book has discussed Kabalistic healing from the perspective of the healer, the one receiving the healing is as important as the one directing the healing process. And while the healer may help the one who is ill to understand the disease, ultimately it is the "healee" who must change the pattern that produced the illness. Healing energies may be very effective in a temporary "remission" of the distortion, but if those patterns producing it are not altered, the distortion will recur in due time.

Those seeking healing must first acknowledge and accept the fact that a distortion or disease either has manifested as a symptom of a higher disharmony or is indicating the need to integrate a certain principle of Divine life. Either through their own awareness or by seeking counseling, they should align the inharmonious manifestation with the quality of energy whose imbalance has produced the pattern's distortion. They should do whatever is indicated, both medically and psychologically, to alleviate the problem, along with seeking the services of a healer to augment and enhance the process necessary to achieve balance. To focus or concentrate on the disease itself will only cause it to intensify. Using every ounce of discipline and intellect possible, an individual should begin to manifest the quality made evident to him, whether it is tolerance, self-worth, right motivation, or selflessness. This is not easy and often requires outside help. One must not think of the disease's eradication in terms of just one lifetime; rather, one should consider the overall plan from a higher perspective. One must accept the fact that it may be necessary for the physical body to die, so that he may begin anew. He must accept this without resentment, becoming aware that the growth experience he can attain from the disease far outweighs the value of a physical vehicle. One should endeavor to understand death, knowing that it is a release of bodily imprisonment when the vehicle is no longer usable.

It is difficult to believe, but nonetheless true, that there are many whose lives are focused around disease. Listen to conversations around you and you will hear discussions regarding illnesses; some people even brag about the severity of their illnesses and describe in great depth their various treatments. In a sense, these individuals have actually identified themselves with the disease, so much so that it becomes the core of their existence. They have given it life!

In his book *Anatomy of an Illness,* Norman Cousins wrote about how he cured his critical illness by watching an endless array of comedy videos. This is an example of diverting conscious

200

attention from a disease to something outside of self. Laughter is one of the highest vibrations. The inner form of laughter is joy, and this joy evidences itself when one devotes oneself to selfless efforts. It is doubtful that comedy films will help everyone, since each individual has a different perception of comedy. But the experience of Norman Cousins does indicate that if attention can be withdrawn from an illness, there is a far greater chance for healing energies, both external and internal, to correct the pattern distortion that produced the illness. To continually direct energy to something strengthens it, while the withdrawal of energy starves it to death.

Both healer and healee must accept the fact that a flow of Divine will directs the being known as man, and they must have absolute faith in that flow, which we can term the will of God. Miracles can and do occur, but one who holds fast to the hope for a miracle is actually bound within his own expectations, restricting movement into balance.

Healer and healee work in partnership. One cannot say "I'm broke, fix me" and expect healing to be effective, especially when the healee is capable of expending his own efforts. We must consider the continuity of life as it has extended from the past and will extend into the future. To live is of far greater importance than to merely exist.

The healee must approach his relationship with the healer with an open mind. Certainly, the wish for every transference of healing energy is for wellness, but focus should be directed to the journey leading to that goal. As stated in the beginning of this book, Divine life is whole, and by adjusting one's life to receive that wholeness, healing occurs. As the consciousness of man continues to evolve, we will see a greater use of vibrational medicine to heal the diseases and distortions of mankind. As each person allows the Tree of Life within himself to grow, then he too will be able to direct its life-will and life-force to others. Kabalistic healers are those who, through the transformative process of the Kabalah, have allowed the Tree within them to grow and are able to direct its healing principles to those in need of them.

BIBLIOGRAPHY

Bailey, Alice. *Esoteric Healing*. New York: Lucis Publishing, 1960.

Besant, Annie. *The Ancient Wisdom*. Adyar, Madras, India: The Theosophical Publishing House, 1939.

Blavatsky, Helena P. *The Secret Doctrine*. Vol. 1. Wheaton, Ill.: Theosophical Publishing House, 1978.

———. *The Secret Doctrine*. Vol. 2. Wheaton, Ill.: Theosophical Publishing House, 1978.

Chambers, Shirley. *Kabalah: A Process of Awakening*. Vol. 1. Atlanta, Ga.: Karin Kabalah Inc., 1992.

———. *Kabalah: A Process of Awakening*. Vol. 2. Atlanta, Ga.: Karin Kabalah Inc., 1992.

———. *Kabalah: A Process of Awakening*. Vol. 3. Atlanta, Ga.: Karin Kabalah Inc., 1992.

Fortune, Dion. *The Mystical Qabalah*. York Beach, Mass.: Samuel Weiser, 1984.

Gray, William G. *Ladder of Lights*. York Beach, Mass.: Samuel Weiser, 1968.

Halevi, Z'ev ben Shimon. *Kabbalah: Tradition of Hidden Knowledge*. New York: Thames and Judson, Inc. 1979.

―――――. *A Kabbalistic Universe*. York Beach, Mass.: Samuel Weiser, 1977.

―――――. *Psychology and Kabbalah*. York Beach, Mass.: Samuel Weiser, 1986.

Hay, Louise. *Heal Your Body*. Carlsbad, Calif.: Hay House, Inc., 1982.

Jung, Carl G. *Man and His Symbols*. New York: Dell Publishing, 1964.

―――――. *Modern Man in Search of a Soul*. Orlando, Fl.: Harcourt Brace and Co., 1933.

―――――. *Symbols of Transformation*. Princeton, N.J.: Princeton University Press, 1956.

Leadbeater, Charles. *The Inner Life*. Wheaton, Ill: Theosophical Publishing House, 1978.

Lofthus, Myra. *A Spiritual Approach to Astrology*. Reno, Nev.: CRCS Publications, 1983.

Love, Jeff. *The Quantum Gods*. New York: Samuel Weiser, 1979.

Manser, Ann. *Pages of Shustah*. St. Petersburg, Fl.: Shustah, Inc., 1974.

Parker, Julia. *The Astrologer's Handbook*. Sebastopol, Calif.: CRSC Publications, 1975.

de Purucker, G. *Studies in Occult Philosophy*. Pasadena, Calif.: Theosophical University Press, 1973.

Scholem, Gershom. *On the Kabbalah and its Symbolism*. New York: Schocken Books, Inc., 1965.

Suares, Carlo. *The Qabala Trilogy: The Cypher of Genesis, The Song of Songs, The Sepher Yetsira*. Boston, Mass.: Shambhala Publications, 1985.

Weil, Andrew. *Spontaneous Healing*. New York: Fawcett Columbine, 1995.

Wilbur, Ken. *No Boundary*. Boston, Mass.: Shambhala Publications, Inc. 1979.

―――――. *The Spectrum of Consciousness*. Wheaton, Ill.: Theosophical Publishing House, 1977.

INDEX

E

F

Force, Pillar of, 16, 17
form, 16, 18, 22, 38, 40, 41
Form, Pillar of, 16, 17

G

Gathas, 3
Geburah, 14, 15, 20, 21, 144,
    145, 168, 176
Geburah of Assiah, 131
Geburah of Yetzirah, 132
Gemara, 6
Genesis, 2, 3, 11, 12, 18, 28, 41,
    73, 79, 102, 128–29
genetic predisposition to disease,
    112, 114–16
    avoiding disease and, 115–16
Gnostics, 7
God
    creative nature of, 39
    as Kether, 172
    as life-will within all existence,
        11
    Worlds of, 33–34, 35
God the Father, World of, 35
God the Mother, World of, 35,
    61
golden yellow, 172, 176
gonorrhea, 122, 123
good, 18
gratitude, expressing, 186
green, 176–77
growth
    balanced continuum of, 39–40
    resistance to, and influenza, 98
    Universal nature and, 43
gut feelings, 142

H

Halakah, 6
harmony, 48, 53, 81
healees
    and healers, 199–202
    recommendations for, 199–200
healer, wounded. See Chiron
healing. See also Kabalistic heal-
        ers; Kabalistic healing
    body's process of, 162, 165
    centering and, 182, 183, 185
    defined, 95
    establishment of harmony and,
        95
    function of, 165
    latent abilities for, 163
    physicians and, 162
    through visualization tech-
        niques, 167, 181
healing energies, 45–46, 108–9.
    See also life-force energy
    Chiron and, 65, 67
    colors, 172–79
    directing, in visualization,
        184–85
    Kabalistic healing and, 159,
        191–98
    levels of mind on Tree of Life
        and, 162–63, 164, 165–69
    Tree of Life and, 162–63
    unconscious mind and, 45–46
health
    harmony and, 53–54
    spiritual awareness and, 100
heart, 143, 144
heart chakra, 97
heart disease, 99, 111, 122
Heikhaloth Books, 4

209

Q

R

S

213

215